Fear

(Illustrated Edition)

By

Angelo Mosso

The Echo Library 2019

Published by

The Echo Library

Echo Library
Unit 22
Horcott Industrial Estate
Horcott Road
Fairford
Glos. GL7 4BX

www.echo-library.com

Please report serious faults in the text to complaints@echo-library.com

ISBN   978-1-40682-041-6

FEAR

BY

ANGELO MOSSO

TRANSLATED FROM THE FIFTH EDITION OF THE ITALIAN
BY
E. LOUGH AND F. KIESOW

AUTHORISED TRANSLATION

LONGMANS, GREEN, AND CO.
LONDON, NEW YORK, AND BOMBAY

1896

3

TO

PROFESSOR ANGELO MOSSO
OF TURIN

from whom both have received many kindnesses of a personal character, and to whom one of us is indebted for furtherance in scientific research, we offer our sincerest thanks, with the assurance that we have looked upon the translation of this splendid little work, as the fulfilment of an agreeable duty.

E. L. and F. K.

August 1895

CONTENTS

ILLUSTRATIONS

FEAR

INTRODUCTION

I

Never shall I forget that evening! From behind the curtains of a glass door I peered into the large amphitheatre crowded with people. It was my first appearance as a lecturer, and most humbly did I repent having undertaken to try my powers in the same hall in which my most celebrated teachers had so often spoken. All I had to do was to communicate the results of some of my investigations into the physiology of sleep, and yet, as the hour drew nearer, stronger waxed within me the fear that I should become confused, lose myself, and finally stand gaping, speechless before my audience. My heart beat violently, its very strings seemed to tighten, and my breath came and went, as when one looks down into a yawning abyss. At last it struck eight. As I cast a last glance at my notes, I became aware, to my horror, that the chain of ideas was broken and the links lost beyond recall. Experiments performed a hundred times, long periods which I had thought myself able to repeat word for word—all seemed forgotten, swept away as though it had never been.

My anguish reached a climax. So great was my perturbation that the recollection of it is dim and shadowy. I remember seeing the usher touch the handle of the door, and that, as he opened it, I seemed to feel a puff of wind in my face; there was a singing in my ears, and then I found myself near a table in the midst of an oppressive silence, as though, after a plunge in a stormy sea, I had raised my head above water and seized hold of a rock in the centre of the vast amphitheatre.

How strange was the sound of my first words! My voice seemed to lose itself in a great wilderness, words, scarce fallen from my lips, to tremble and die away. After a few sentences jerked out almost mechanically, I perceived that I had already finished the introduction to my speech, and discovered with dismay that memory had played me false just at that point where I had thought myself most sure; but there was now no turning back, and so, in great confusion, I proceeded. The hall seemed enveloped in mist. Slowly the cloud began to lift, and here and there in the crowd I could distinguish benevolent, friendly faces, and on these I fixed my gaze, as a man struggling with the waves clings to a floating spar. I could discern, too, the attentive countenances of eager listeners, holding a hand to their ear as though unwilling to lose a single word, and nodding occasionally in token of affirmation. And lastly, I saw myself in this semicircle, alone, humbled, discouraged, dejected—like a sinner at confession. The first greatest emotional disturbance was over; but my throat was parched, my cheeks burned, my breath came in gasps, my voice was strained and trembling. The harmony of the period was often interrupted in the middle by a rapid inspiration, or painfully drawn out, as the chest was compressed to lend force to the last words of a sentence. But to my joy, in spite of all, the ideas began to unfold of their own accord, following each other in regular order along the magic thread to which I blindly clung without a backward glance, and which was to lead me out of the labyrinth. Even the trembling of the hands, which had made me shake the instruments and drawings I had from time to time to exhibit, ceased at last. A heaviness crept over my whole body, the muscles seemed to stiffen, and my knees shook.

Towards the end I felt the blood begin to circulate again. A few minutes passed of which I remember nothing save a great anxiety. My trembling voice had assumed the conclusive tone adopted at the close of a speech. I was perspiring, exhausted, my strength was failing; I glanced at the tiers of seats, and it seemed to me that they were slowly opening in front of me, like the jaws of a monster ready to devour me as soon as the last word should re-echo within its throat.

II

He who one day will write a book on the physiology of the orator will render a great service to society—to us who have to pay so dearly for 'that extravagant idolatry of ourselves' which incites us to speak in public. But such a work must be a complete treatise, a mirror in which each might see himself and learn to what ridicule he exposes himself, what punishment awaits him, when he mounts the rostrum uncalled for and untried. Each must see himself with pallid cheeks, perturbed, distorted countenance, suffering from that unhealthy excitement which, like a storm of emotion, breaks out in trembling. Before entering the lists let each feel the oppression on the chest, the cough, the compression of the bladder, the loss of appetite, the unquenchable thirst, the dizziness which will blind him; and lastly, let each endure in advance all the innumerable gradations of pitying sympathy awakened in the audience by his own timidity.

We can better understand the influence of the emotions on the organism if we consider the long novitiate, the unwearying efforts and the countless trials of even the greatest orators before they attained to self-control, and to the simple end of preserving before the public the same intonation, gestures, and persuasive force which are natural to them when in the company of their friends or the retirement of the family circle.

I have seen men of brilliant intelligence standing rigid, their arms hanging at their sides like recruits, their features distorted and their eyes fixed on the ground, stammering and grinding out their speech, so as to move one to pity. Others, known to their intimates as jovial anecdotists, make one turn away one's eyes in compassion when, on important occasions, they stop short in the middle of a sentence, gasp, repeat the same word four or five times, struggling for utterance, and at last stand still open-mouthed, clutching the table or their watch-chain, as though in search of an anchor of salvation. Others, again, go to a banquet and succeed in damping all gaiety.

At the very beginning it is evident that food is swallowed with difficulty, their speech lies heavy on their heart, they are nervous and tortured by the fear that their memory may leave them in the lurch. One pities them when at last they rise pale and trembling, then speak confusedly, jerkily, swaying to and fro with wide-open eyes, as though stupefied with agitation.

A former master of mine, once professor of sacred rhetoric at the Athenæum of Turin, could, at the beginning of a nervous affection, only speak sitting, owing to the excessive trembling of his legs; and at last he was obliged to renounce the triumphs which his masterly and enviable gift of eloquence procured him, as he was unable, after having concluded his speech, either to rise, to descend from the cathedra, or to walk.

But why does the simple fact that we are standing before the public produce such disquietude within us? Why is it followed by such a far-reaching disturbance of the organic functions? We say it is the nerves, the brain, anxiety, the physical nature of man which we cannot control. But there is confusion also in our ideas. What is this much-praised force of will, this power of the soul which makes us so bold when alone and yet so cowardly before the eyes of a few people?

I confess the problem is difficult, and I believe the easiest way to a partial solution is to analyse without prejudice what we all know about cerebral activity, and to see what physiologists have discovered in studying the emotions and the physical phenomena of thought.

III

Before, however, entering the field of experimental physiology, I allow myself the following remarks. In strict justice the names of many physiologists should be repeatedly mentioned, but I prefer to do so only from time to time, as I fear the interruption of the sentence by names and notes might be tiresome to those whose eye is unaccustomed to the perusal of scientific books, nor do I think there are many who would be curious to know the paternity of every assertion I shall make use of. In order, however, that no undeserved merit may be ascribed to me, I shall, without further ceremony, write in the first person only when an experience or an idea of my own is to be communicated, so that, if I shall be at fault, science may not be held responsible for a personal error.

The first really important book on the physiology of the passions was written by Descartes, the great restorer of science, who, with his prodigious force of intellect, embraced all branches of knowledge, and was at once mathematician, physicist, and physiologist. His is the honour of having shown that the old Aristotelian philosophy, then prevalent in the schools, had never solved one of the problems respecting life. In the treatise upon 'The Passions of the Soul,' the following words appear in a section in which he investigates the manner in which the passions are excited: 'If the appearance of an animal is very strange and frightful—that is, if it has much resemblance with those things which were originally hurtful to the body, it will excite in the mind the passion of fear, then of boldness or of horror, according to the different temperaments of the body or the force of the soul, and according as one has been able or not to provide one's self with the means of defence, or of flight from those dangerous things with which the present impression has points of resemblance. This in some men disposes the brain in such a manner that the spirits, excited by the image and formed in the pineal gland (or central part of the brain), pass thence, partly to the nerves which serve to turn the body and move the legs in flight, and partly to those nerves which enlarge and contract the valves of the heart, or stimulate the other parts, whence the blood is sent to them in such a manner that this blood, otherwise elaborated, sends spirits to the brain capable of fomenting and increasing the passion of fear; that is, they are able to keep open or reopen the pores of the brain which conduct them to the nerves.[1]

No one before Descartes had had so simple a conception of the mechanism by which the involuntary movements accompanying the emotions are produced, and he it is who laid the foundations of the physiological study of the mind. Two centuries and a half have already passed, and his work still remains a monument worthy of all admiration. Science has advanced so greatly that perhaps no one now who wished to learn the elements of physiology would study his treatise on man, and yet none who know the history of science but are moved by those marvellous pages out of which breathes that spirit of innovation which has fertilised the science of centuries. Malebranche relates that when he first took up the treatise—'L'homme et la formation du fœtus,' by Descartes—the new ideas it stirred up within him gave him a pleasure so intense, and so filled him with admiration, that his heart palpitated and he was obliged to pause from time to time.

Other two no less celebrated names must also be mentioned here, on account of the strictly scientific character they have given to the study of the emotions. These are Herbert Spencer and Charles Darwin. Next to these stands Paolo Mantegazza, with his celebrated researches on pain and his book on physiognomy and mimicry, dedicated to 'Charles Darwin, who, by his immortal work on the expression of the emotions, opened up a limitless horizon to the science of the future.' The homage of the illustrious Italian physiologist is worthy of the great English master and philosopher. Darwin was a man of genius and at the same time one of the greatest masters of the popular style of authorship. His force lies in the caution with which he made statements and drew conclusions, thus avoiding all absolute formulæ, and this will always make him an incomparable model. Dogmatism, that worm which gnaws and sterilises mediocre minds, which corrupts the rationality of the many—dogmatism, that plague of science, had no hold on him, Darwin knew it not. He candidly shows the public the gaps in science, criticises himself unmercifully, and does not hesitate to point out the defects in doctrines he himself propounded. In reading his books one is

---

[1] Œuvres de Descartes, *Les passions de l'âme*, xxxvi.

inclined to think that he was continually haunted by the fear of being misunderstood by readers insufficiently educated for the comprehension of deeper scientific questions. He was so careful, so temperate in his assertions, so cautious in his inductions, that in his book, 'The Expression of the Emotions,' which, in my opinion, is one of the less excellent of his works, he leaves not one point on which one can conscientiously contradict him, by taxing him with an error.

And if we are able now to add to his discoveries and to correct some of the judgments in his works, it is only thus because science marches onward with such giant strides that we, although we were his contemporaries, belong even now to a later age, as the context of this work will more clearly show. The theory of evolution will always remain the foundation-stone of modern science, but certain principles formulated by Spencer and Darwin will be modified as our knowledge of the adaptation of organs to their functions increases.

IV

Darwin attributed, I think, too much importance to the will considered as the cause of expression. We younger physiologists are more mechanical; we examine the organism more minutely, and it is in the structure of the organs that we seek the reasons of their functions.

I shall here give an example of this different way in which I have explained a few phenomena.

Rabbits are, as is well known, extremely timid animals, and it is remarkable that no other blushes and grows pale so easily as the rabbit. The changes in circulation produced by psychical impressions and by the emotions are more observable in the ears than in the face, as is indeed the case with many men. In Northern Italy, after someone has received a vigorous scolding, I have heard the popular expression used: 'He caught it hot enough to make his ears turn red.' In the middle of the auricle of the rabbit's ear there is an artery, running from the base to the summit, which ramifies and winds in such a manner as to form two veins on the edge of the auricle. In 1854, Moritz Schiff observed that this artery showed alternate movements of contraction and expansion, not corresponding to the systole and diastole of the heart. If one looks at the rabbit's ear against the light, from time to time one sees the artery decrease in diameter, until at last it quite disappears, then it increases again, and, as it swells, it expands all its branches, so that the whole ear becomes of a vivid red and also warmer. This fulness of blood in the ear lasts a few seconds, then artery and branches contract and the redness gradually dies away. Schiff called this artery an accessory heart, because he imagined that the contractions and expansions observed by him in the vessels of the ear were to promote a better circulation of blood in the ear of the rabbit, just as the heart does for the rest of the body.

In repeating Schiff's observations I used certain precautions which others would perhaps have thought superfluous. Instead of watching the rabbit while holding it in my hands, I thought to spare it all emotion, by enabling myself to observe the ears without its becoming aware of the fact. For this purpose I had a cage made in such a manner that it fitted exactly into the inside frame of a window, and whereas it was impossible for the rabbits to look into the room, I could watch quite easily, without being seen, through a few holes in the cage. By means of this simple arrangement I could observe the rabbits at my leisure, and study their habits while they were quiet, without a suspicion that they were being noticed. The first time that I so watched them, I saw, to my surprise, that the ears were no longer so red as when the animals were startled by feeling themselves seized and held fast in my hands on the table. The rapid movements of dilatation and contraction in the blood-vessels of the ear, the sudden blushing and loss of colour so characteristic of the timidity of these animals, were no longer observable. The artery of the ear remained dilated and of a vivid red for a long time, often for hours. I noticed this especially in summer, when the animals were uniformly tranquil. A state of absolute repose, however, is not always accompanied by an expansion of the blood-vessels. All rabbits have not ears equally red or pale at the same time and under the same conditions. A similar circumstance may be noticed at any time in the faces of men. Young rabbits blush more easily than old ones. Often while watching the buck and doe with the young ones, one could see the ruddy ears of the latter turn pale every now and then, while the former, like old people with us, remained calm and had pale ears. But even amongst the young ones of the same litter, one finds considerable differences in the facility for blushing.

At the market I chose those animals that blushed most easily and frequently, just as the slave-dealer picks out for the harem those women who charm by blushing more vividly than the others. If one studies attentively the loss of colour in the ears of a rabbit when perfectly quiet, one can nearly always discover the cause in some external circumstance. Often while the animal has red ears and is breathing quietly, one notices a sudden change in the rhythm of respiration; the rabbit lifts its head, looks around, or sniffs; a contraction of the blood-vessels follows, and the ears become pale. After a few minutes, if nothing happens, the ear becomes red again. Any noise causes renewed pallor. A whistle, a cry, a sound of any kind, the bark of a dog, a sunbeam suddenly penetrating into the cage, the shadow of a swiftly passing cloud, the flight of a distant bird, each suffices to produce a rapid loss of colour in the ears, shortly followed by a more vivid flush. We may therefore maintain that the circulation of blood in the ears reflects the psychic condition of the animal, and that nothing takes place either in itself or in its surroundings without immediately acting upon these blood-vessels.

Thus the fact observed by Schiff receives confirmation, but the explanation which I give of it differs from his. The dilatation and contraction of the arteries in the rabbit's ear can no longer be compared to the movements of an accessory heart, and, in my opinion, correspond to the colour or pallor of the human face. In this manner the phenomenon is deprived of the exceptional character with which it was introduced into science, and takes its place amongst those observable in man and nearly all animals.

We may see the same phenomenon noticeable in the rabbit's ear, in the cock's comb and wittles; during emotion the fleshy protuberances and the skin on the neck of the turkey distinctly blush and grow pale, and in men and dogs not only the face but also the feet are subject to these changes of colour.

These things were unknown owing to insufficient observation. It was thought that animals did not blush, because the blood-vessels of their skin lie concealed under hair, feathers, or scales, and because the epidermis is less transparent and the pigment cells more abundant in the lower layers of the skin. And so blushing was deemed a privilege of man, which, however, is not the case. It suffices to study the face of the rabbit attentively in order to see that it is very sensitive, even to the slightest impressions. If one looks carefully at the nostrils and lips, considerable variations in the colour may be observed, corresponding to those occurring at the same time in the blood-vessels of the ear. These phenomena became so familiar to me during my study of rabbits, that I needed only observe the muzzle of the animal, and more particularly the tip, in order to know at once whether the ears were at that moment pale or red. This certainty was in part due to the alteration in the rhythm of breathing and in the movement of the nostrils produced by the slightest emotion, as also in man.

V

Many may regret that such a characteristic difference between man and the other animals should be effaced, and that we should try in cold blood to prove that what is most noble, beautiful, and human in our countenance, we have in common with the brutes. But we console ourselves with the reflection that poetry, enthusiasm, inspiration and passion rise again under new and stronger forms in the contemplation of reality, that in the search after truth there lies a fascination which beautifies and ennobles the human intelligence, and that sentiment is never extinguished by any advance of science.

To-day, when the experimental method is spreading so rapidly, it behoves us physiologists to be humble and to ask for hospitality in the studio of the artist, in the libraries of men of letters, in the drawing-rooms of cultured people, in order to diffuse the elementary principles of our science. The time has come when we must throw off our professorial robes, tie on our aprons, roll up our sleeves, and begin the vivisection of the human heart according to scientific methods.

Let the artist no longer confine himself to a blind imitation of nature, to a perpetual reproduction on canvas, in marble, or in books of the phenomena and forms of life; he must know the why and wherefore of things, completely or in part, the connection between cause and effect; he must convince himself that nothing is the result of chance and that there is a reason behind every phenomenon. Blushing—that ideal token of innocence and purity—is no accidental fact; it was not given to man as a sign of nobility, nor as a mirror to reflect the agitation of his heart; it is a fact rendered necessary by bodily functions and which the will can neither produce nor suppress. It is simply caused by the structure of our vital machine, by the activity of the blood-vessels in all organs and in all animals.

Darwin believed, on the contrary, that it was a phenomenon produced by means of the will. I consider it advisable to quote here in full the explanation which he gives of blushing, as no other naturalist made it the object of such special study, and because his hypothesis is at variance with the facts of my observation.

'Men and women, and especially the young, have always valued, in a high degree, their personal appearance, and have likewise regarded the appearance of others. The face has been the chief object of attention, though, when man aboriginally went naked, the whole surface of his body would have been attended to. Our self-attention is excited almost exclusively by the opinion of others, for no person living in absolute solitude would care about his appearance. Everyone feels blame more acutely than praise. Now, whenever we know, or suppose, that others are depreciating our personal appearance, our attention is strongly drawn toward ourselves, more especially to our faces. The probable effect of this will be, as has just been explained, to excite into activity that part of the sensorium which receives the sensory nerves of the face; and this will react through the vaso-motor system on the facial capillaries. By frequent reiteration during numberless generations, the process will have become so habitual, in association with the belief that others are thinking of us, that even a suspicion of their depreciation suffices to relax the capillaries, without any conscious thought about our faces. With some sensitive persons it is enough even to notice their dress to produce the same effect. Through the force, also, of association and inheritance our capillaries are relaxed, whenever we know, or imagine, that anyone is blaming, though in silence, our actions, thoughts, or character; and, again, when we are highly praised.'

'On this hypothesis we can understand how it is that the face blushes more than any other part of the body.' 'Of all expressions, blushing seems to be the most strictly human.' 'But it does not seem possible that any animal, until its mental powers had been developed to an equal or nearly equal degree with those of man, would have closely considered and been sensitive about its own personal appearance. Therefore we may conclude that blushing originated at a very late period in the long line of our descent.'[2]

I hold that this explanation of blushing is no longer tenable, and I think that perhaps Darwin himself would have accepted mine, since it seems to me truer, more in correspondence with the theory of evolution, more Darwinian, if I may be allowed the expression.

But why do we blush? some will ask, who insist on penetrating to the root of things. Why, under certain conditions, does the blood flow more abundantly into the rabbit's ear and the human face? The answer to this question will be better understood when I have shown that the brain also becomes redder after an emotion. For the

---

[2] Charles Darwin: *The Expression of the Emotions*, pp. 345 and 364. London, 1872.

maintenance of life it is necessary that a dilatation of the blood-vessels should take place in all those organs in which a disturbance occurs. We all know that when our hand has been firmly squeezed, or when we have received a blow or contusion, the skin reddens at once. This change in the circulation is indispensable, for the more copious flow of blood to that part which has suffered an arrest of nutrition serves to renew the vital processes and to repair the damage caused by the injury. The same phenomena appear in the brain under psychic conditions. Emotion occasions greater energy in the chemical processes of the brain; there is a modification in the nutrition of the cells, the nervous force is more rapidly consumed, and therefore the expansion of the blood-vessels of head and brain tend, by a more abundant supply of blood, to preserve the activity of the nerve-centres.

It is in the tissues, in the properties of the living substances which constitute the vital machine, that we must seek the reasons of numerous phenomena which Darwin deduced from external causes, natural selection or environment. We shall endeavour to confine within much narrower limits the effects of chance, will, and accident, which play such an important part in Darwin's theory. Nothing is the result of a creative force serving a premeditated end; organisms have formed and changed themselves through causes exclusively mechanical. Work perfects organisms, and the operative parts undergo, through their own activity, far-reaching modifications, which render their structure still more perfect.

CHAPTER I

HOW THE BRAIN WORKS

I

Before beginning the study of the nerve-centres I shall remind the reader of a few very simple facts, which, doubtless, he already knows, but which, recalled, will render more apparent the part taken by the body in the functions of the mind.

In order to know how the brain works, it is sufficient to recall the pictures and visions which pass before us when we are absent-minded. How curious it is when the mind sets out on its fanciful wanderings! when, unconsciously, we leave the everyday world behind us and stand motionless, with open eyes, seeing and hearing nothing.

How often in the quiet of our study, while reading a book, have we not seen the words gradually fade one into another, until we found ourselves as though enveloped in a cloud, far away amid the recollections of childhood or the hopes of the future! And what wonderful forms grow out of the flames, the logs, and the sparks glowing under the ashes, when we draw close to the fire in lonely evenings!

It is an actual relief to many, this repose of attention, this extinction of the will which steals over us in the midst of life's troubles, lifting the burden of care and allowing us to contemplate quietly the curious spectacle which, when left to itself, the brain at work presents. How rapidly things and thoughts are transformed, melting into each other without order, aim, or pause! How easily we glide by winding paths through time and space, while in endless succession new horizons and new countries rise before us! What airy phantoms look down from the clouds above, what voices and harmonies strike the ear in the waterfalls of the brooks, what living pictures peer at us from amongst the flowers and grasses on the bank! Then suddenly a flood of memories rushes over us and leaves us confused, bewildered, as it rolls on again to the dim horizon of consciousness. And in this rushing flood of thoughts and forms we see the familiar faces of those whom the grave seems to give back to us, and we hasten to meet them with smiling lips or with tears in our eyes.

II

And yet these are nought but dreams of the waking mind. Even when the force of attention and the energy of thought are greater, we still are carried away by the wilful, untamable current of cerebral activity; because the will can do nothing within the domain of the imagination, and because the brain is no slave who will obey our very nod. Who does not remember the painful and useless endeavours made to rid oneself of an annoying thought and that incapacity for mental work which afflicts us, without our knowing whence it came? How often have we sat for hours at the desk, with idle pen, our head in our hands, unable to wrest even one thought from the mind which we dared transmit to paper! How depressed we are on those days when the sources of the mind seem dried up, when we torture ourselves in vain, ransacking our brains and finding nothing but fragments, crumbs of thought which we reject angrily as worthless refuse!

We must resign ourselves. We feel ourselves humbled as though the door of our own house had been shut in our face. It is of no use to be sad and annoyed; even if we give way to furious passion, it does not help us. We stand behind a high wall which we cannot break down. An English physiologist compared the thinking man to a simple engine-driver. He does not move the trains, neither does he determine their departure or their stoppage, he merely guides their movement, directing them first in one direction then in another.

The brain is perpetually at work, and it is impossible for the mind to embrace its activities in every part. The greater the attention is in one part, the more vague is the knowledge which we have of contiguous parts, the less vivid are the impressions which the senses transmit from the outside world. We need only recall the well-known example of Archimedes who was killed by a Roman soldier during the siege of Syracuse, while he stood in calm contemplation of some geometrical figures.

The whole of our brain is never at work at one time; now it is the one half, then the other which is in action.

When looking at the sky or at a wall in a uniform light with only one eye, I found that the field of vision changed alternately from light to dark. This does not depend upon the eye but upon the brain, because unconsciously we use first one eye then the other; and, in the same way, the two hemispheres of the brain do not work simultaneously, sometimes it is the one sometimes the other which is in a state of activity. A French general had lost one half of his brain from a wound which clove the skull. He recovered and retained his intelligence and gaiety, but he used soon to grow tired during conversation and could only continue any intense mental work for a few minutes at a time.

There are many philosophers who maintain that a considerable portion of our cerebral activity is purely automatic, so that our mind is often in operation without our being conscious of it. When an idea, says Maudsley,[3] disappears from the horizon of consciousness, it need not vanish totally, but may remain, as it were, latent or veiled, continuing by its movements to awaken, to give rise to, other ideas without our being aware of this activity. But when our consciousness is unexpectedly drawn off from its work, or roused by something which had before occupied it, then we catch the idea at work.

This opinion is rendered probable by a few phenomena which I observed during my studies of the circulation of the blood in the brain, and we may easily convince

_____

[3] Maudsley: *The Physiology of Mind*, p. 305. London, 1876.

ourselves also, if we reflect, how often, quite unexpectedly, names and events occur to us when we were least thinking of them, and which we were unable to recall for a long time and in spite of wearisome efforts, when we wished to do so. And we all know that we are unable to fall asleep at will, so little mastery have we over our thoughts. We direct our minds first to this object then to that, in order to draw it away from that which occupies it and keeps us awake. We try to suppress an idea which torments us by calling other ideas to our assistance in ousting it, and often wait powerless for the coming of that silent oblivion and calm of mind which alone can give us rest.

If, in the moments preceding sleep, when the mind is comparatively quiet, we make an effort to fix our thoughts on something, we notice how they vacillate, disappearing and reappearing, as though we were in a boat and our heads were lifted from time to time above the waves. Even when awake we find ourselves only too often in this humble bark in which every puff of wind drives us far from the shore we wish to reach, when impetuous currents of thought prevent our entering the haven, or when the waves open to plunge us into unfathomable depths out of which we can see no horizon.

III

But in order better to see the link which binds the substance of our organism to the activity of thought, the correlation between the nutrition of the body and the mental state, or, as one is accustomed to say, the relation between body and soul, let us carefully notice what takes place when a number of friends are assembled at table.

After a few cheerful remarks made by the most jovial as they take their places, a certain gloom spreads over the company. One might almost think only a few were sociably inclined. Someone attempts to break the ice, but it is a failure; one feels that the conversation is forced, jerky, altogether wanting in sparkle. Little by little the guests brighten up. A hum ensues, then a confused buzz, like the tuning of the instruments of an orchestra, which rapidly increases in pitch, as though each were trying to make his voice heard above his neighbour's. It seems as though something in their brains had been loosened and the vocal cords had gradually got into working order. At dessert even the more taciturn, if they have done full justice to the banquet, pour forth an unceasing stream of conversation. Moody faces become smiling, and melancholy gives place to gaiety. The cross-fire of talk, the hot discussions, the frequent bursts of laughter, the lively play of feature, the witty interruptions, the excited gesticulations, all show a hundredfold increase of vital action.

And from the glowing faces, the sparkling eyes, we know that the blood is rushing in abundance to the brain. The tongue is loosed, ideas accumulate in the mind, as though some kind hand had set the rusty wheels of thought in motion and poured oil on the hinges of the vocal mechanism.

There is no need to say more. We have all experienced this transformation which takes place in the work of the brain. It enters on another phase when the wine begins to circulate. If we had not already met the guests on similar social occasions, we should be greatly surprised at their metamorphosis, and feel constrained to correct previous misconceptions of their character. Men, whom I had always thought silent and cold, I have seen, to my amazement, carrying on the most daring discussions with brilliant fluency, and rebutting sarcasms with such promptitude and success as to earn them loud applause. Other timid ones, known to all as slow, tiresome, clumsy talkers, find in the wine-glass a sparkling vivacity, a flow of speech which makes them more agreeable; nor do they hesitate to propose toasts and drink to the health of each of the guests. They rise, glass in hand, finding a witty word for each and showering compliments on all sides. Men, calm and sedate, in whom none suspected a poetic soul, are capable of rising and improvising verses, and we are full of admiration at their skill, and at the harmonious grace of rhythm, metaphor, and rhyme.

Each one feels something like inspiration within him, as though warmed by the quickening pulse of life.

But let us leave the joyous company: so far as our psychological study is concerned, we have already lingered too long, and it would be superfluous to follow them as they leave, in order to see how confident, kind, and courageous they have all become.

The next day each will resume his own character and his own business. If it happens that one of the guests meets another in the street, they smile as they shake hands, and words which are a revelation are heard: 'We were a lively party last night, eh? I scarcely recognised *you*, and as for some others, there was no keeping them quiet!'

IV

The analysis of memory better than anything else shows us the connection between the various parts of the brain which enter into activity in order to provide us with the elements that form speech.

We must distinguish two kinds of memory:

1. The fixation of impressions, whether these be images, or representations of movements, words, sounds or sensations.

2. The re-awakening of these impressions as recollection.

The phenomena of memory remain quite incomprehensible if we do not admit their intimate connection with physical changes of the nerve substance. An external impression acting upon receptive nerve-cells is retained by them permanently, as though it were photographed, if it be allowable to explain the unknown by a comparison with the known. It is the blood which carries those substances to the brain which are necessary to the functions of memory. Attention cannot be developed in all its intensity without causing considerable alterations in the circulation. Now when we are absent-minded, images leave no lasting impression on the memory, as no provision is then made by the physical changes in the organism accompanying attention for a more rapid circulation of blood in the cerebral hemispheres.

The old notion that the brain was a storehouse in which each idea had its nook where it might stay till needed, is truer than it appears. Modern science has proved that the matter is much more complicated than one thinks. It suffices that the blood should coagulate in the artery which carries it to some convolution, or that a tumour should destroy a part of the brain, for us to lose, as it were, a province of memory.

Let us first consider verbal memory. That region of the brain in which it is placed is, generally speaking, the parietal region of the left side; so that anyone who has had a blow on the temple at that side nearly always loses his speech, although he still remembers things and can pronounce their names when they are repeated to him by others, a sufficient proof that the movements of the tongue are not impeded. Sometimes it happens that a person in this condition looks in the dictionary for the missing word, in order to recover the pronunciation of it.

In learning a language, we believe that certain cells undertake functions which they did not before possess, that connections with other cells are established, like very intricate nets in which the impressions of nouns and verbs, the graphic representations of ideas and words, are collected. As we exercise ourselves in the language, the blood carries new elements to these cells, and the greater our attention, the stronger become the impressions. Oxidation does not destroy the impression once received, but it weakens it. If we have had no practice for some years in speaking a language, we meet with great difficulties, our communications being made in set, stiff words; but after a few days one regains the former fluency.

We might quote cases in which, through illness, a man has completely forgotten a language, recovering it as health returned. Others have forgotten several languages in the order of succession in which they had learnt them, regaining them later in the inverse order to that of acquisition.

When groping in the dim recesses of memory, we always perceive that there are associations and intimate connections amongst the phenomena of thought. The blood, making its way into certain parts of the brain, is like the light of a torch penetrating subterranean passages, on the walls of which are painted pictures of things we know. Often the blood-vessels do not yield, and we then wander in vain in that labyrinth, retracing our steps, roaming hither and thither, until suddenly we see an opening, and what we were seeking appears unexpectedly before us. The supposition that we here have to do with an effect of the blood, an expansion or contraction of the vessels, and with phenomena of nutrition, seems to be strengthened by the circumstance that sometimes, in consequence of violent emotion, a succession of things which before seemed totally forgotten suddenly reappears in our memory.

The link between physical phenomena and phenomena of memory is more apparent during fatigue and the refreshing state of repose. Memory may fail entirely from anæmia, from poisoning by narcotics, innutrition of the brain, and in old age; for we all know how much better we remember the events of our youth than those of later occurrence.

Men who have had wounds or contusions on the head have been known to forget that they had children; authors have forgotten even the titles of their works; but as soon as the fever had passed, or the wound healed, they regained their memory. Others, during a fever, have related events and remembered names which they had quite forgotten previously, and which they were unable to recall after recovery.

CHAPTER II

REFLEX ACTION AND THE FUNCTIONS OF THE SPINAL CORD

I

Until 1820 physiologists believed that all nerves had the same functions; that is, that all were sensory.

We can scarcely picture the confusion in the mind of anyone studying the nerves of the face when, besides those destined to the organs of smell, sight, and hearing, he would notice two other large nerves—the Trigeminus and Facialis—passing off separately from the brain and spinal marrow, and which, with a double ramification of filaments, cover all superficial and underlying parts of the face; and again, when he saw the three nerves of various origin which go to the tongue, the four which are distributed in the throat, and finally, in the midst of this net of nerves, thick bundles of fine filaments and ganglia of which the origin was untraceable.

It was an English physiologist, Charles Bell, who solved this problem by showing that the most important nerves of the face, with the exception of the special sensory nerves, are confined to two. If one of these nerves, called the trigeminal, be cut through, every trace of sensibility immediately disappears from the corresponding side of the face; if the other, the facial nerve, be severed, sensibility remains, but the face completely loses the power of movement, there is no longer any contraction of the muscles or change of expression in the face.

I quote Charles Bell's own words, since these two simple experiments still form the base of the physiology of the nervous system.

'If we cut the division of the fifth nerve which goes to the lips of an ass, we deprive the lips of sensibility; so when the animal presses the lips to the ground, and against the oats lying there, it does not feel them, and consequently there is no effort made to gather them. If, on the other hand, we cut the seventh nerve where it goes to the lips, the animal feels the oats, but it can make no effort to gather them, the power of muscular motion being cut off by the division of the nerve.'[4]

The same takes place in the hand, the legs, and in all other parts of the body, which, according as the one or the other set of nerves is injured, feel but cannot move, or move and do not feel.

In the ordinary circumstances of life no one becomes aware of these two fundamental properties of the nervous system, or at least we do not reflect that there are two distinct apparatus: the nerves which make us feel, and the nerves which cause movement. The intimate connection between these in the nerve centres and at the

---

[4] Ch. Bell: *Anatomy and Physiology of the Human Body*, v. ii., p. 394. London, 1826.

surface of the body renders special methods necessary to separate them, and allow them to act independently of each other.

Claude Bernard, the greatest of French physiologists, and one of the most agreeable and successful authors who have ever popularised science, showed how these two elements may be dissociated by introducing certain poisons into the blood, which kill the finest ramifications of the nerves in the most inaccessible parts of the organism.

If one scratches the skin of a dog with a poisoned arrow, like those used in war by certain savage tribes of America, the animal succumbs in less than a quarter of an hour. This terrible poison, called *curari*, destroys the motor nerves, but produces no change in the intelligence, and the functions of the sensory nerves. The dog scarcely notices the slight puncture on the skin and continues to walk about the room; but in a short time the hind-legs become stiff, one can see that they no longer obey the will; the posterior part of the body sways and falls. The animal rises and stumbles; then the fore-legs fail and the dog stands still. If we call him, or pat him, he responds with movements of the head, the ears, the eyes, and by wagging his tail. Soon however he cannot lift his head and lies stretched out, breathing quietly, as though reposing at his ease. On being called, he moves his eyes and feebly wags his tail, without any manifestation of pain. At last the respiratory muscles cease to act and life ebbs out without a single convulsive movement, and for a few moments sensibility and intelligence are still distinguishable in the fixed and glassy eye. It is like a corpse that perceives and understands everything going on around it, without being able to move, retaining sentiment and will but having no means of manifesting them.

II

In an investigation which I made with Professor E. Guareschi[5] into the effect of cadaveric venom, we found that all substances which slowly destroy the organism must produce phenomena analogous to those of curari, since the motor nerves, according to our researches, have less vitality than the sensory.

In order to be convinced of this fact, it suffices to take a rabbit and stop the circulation in its hind-legs. Placed on the ground, after a few seconds the animal cannot move its hind-legs, but if one presses them it squeaks and tries to escape with the aid of its fore-legs, dragging after it the hinder part of its body, which remains paralysed for a few moments. A sudden anæmia can therefore destroy motility but leave sensibility uninjured.

When life is slowly ebbing, when the circulation gradually slackens and the death-agony is prolonged, I believe that there is always a point of time in which, with the exception of the respiratory and cardiac muscles, all others are already paralysed, in which all is dead but the sensory nerves.

---

[5] 'Les Ptomaïnes.' *Archives italiennes de Biologie*, ii. p. 367; iii. p. 241.

The hand, which with a last effort has been laid in blessing on our head, has sunk back on the coverlet never to be raised again, never to move the fingers which still feel the pressure of the farewell clasp; but the fixed eye still sees the shadows of the loved ones bending down to press tearful kisses on the brow, and when the last breath has fled, the mother still hears the despairing cry of her children and can no longer respond even by a look.

III

We have therefore two sorts of nerves: of sensibility and of movement. Let us now try to form a correct notion of an involuntary or reflex movement, which I shall illustrate by the following example.

Let us imagine a large house of which the entrance is at some distance from the street door. A bell is fixed inside, the wire of which, after passing through various holes, terminates in a handle near the outer door. When some one comes and pulls the handle the bell rings, and the maid opens the door by pulling at the cord inside the house. This series of actions represents what physiologists call a reflex movement. The maid is a nerve-centre, the bell-wire a sensory nerve, and the cord which opens the door a motor nerve. In the organism we see muscles or glands instead of the door, but the mechanism is similar. Just as the door-bell rings a hundred times a day on all imaginable occasions without our needing to open the door, and without the maid coming first to our study to ask what she must do; so we have in our nervous system two distinct parts: the maid, represented by the spinal cord, and the master, by the brain.

Let us now see what happens when the master is not at home, or what an animal does when its head is cut off, and only the spinal cord is left. We shall see here, too, that the more liberty the master gives to the maid, the more arrogant she grows, at last lording it over the master himself.

A decapitated frog does not die immediately; it may move for days, and if deprived of the brain only remains alive for some time.

We will consider the more usual case, namely, that of a frog of which the head has been completely cut off with a pair of scissors. The animal shivers and writhes for a few moments, then it stops, and would remain motionless if it were kept under a glass cover in a damp atmosphere, where nothing would irritate the skin. But if we touch its leg or put a drop of vinegar upon it, the animal tries at once to escape and to remove the disturbing agent from the surface of its body. If we put a drop of vinegar on the left leg it tries to wipe it off with the right, and *vice versa*. But if we cut off one of the legs or bind it fast, and then put a drop of vinegar on the other leg which is at liberty, the frog makes use of this same leg to rub away the drop.

At first sight this seems to be an act of intelligence. It may be maintained that it is done by choice, but we cannot say that this activity requires the guidance of the intelligence. A dog of which the spinal cord has been severed and a sleeping man make the same movements.

Neither must it be thought that these movements are only to be found in frogs and the lower animals. We shall see that in man also they perform all the most indispensable vital functions without the co-operation of the brain. Fontana, one of the most celebrated Italian physiologists, discovered, as early as the middle of the last century, that one could decapitate rabbits and guinea-pigs without causing their immediate death. And he also found that if care were taken by previously binding the most important arteries; so that the animal should not lose too much blood, and if the respiration were sustained artificially by means of bellows, it could live for some time, and show itself sensitive to external stimuli.[6]

IV

If we could hear the soliloquies of the man who is writing a book, many, I think, would renounce for ever the pleasure of setting the printing press in motion. It would be a curious experience, if one could read between the lines the tale of discouragement, uncertainty, trouble, and know the repeated struggles by which some difficulty was overcome, a passage was composed, a clause or a sentence written. In scientific works it would be seen that the most frequent interruptions and exclamations arise always from doubt, and the anxiety which torments an author of not making his meaning clear.

There is no remedy. He who wishes to explain a scientific subject in a clear and simple way must stop from time to time; he must come out of himself and take his reader's place, forget all he knows in order to listen impartially to his own voice, and to judge if what he has said may be easily understood. And this I shall do, but the reader must not be repulsed by the first difficulties: our first steps cost the greatest effort. In order to comprehend the physical nature of man, and to know how this exquisite machinery of ours works, we must first examine attentively some of the most important organs which are constantly at work in our nervous system. It is in science as in the study of languages, one must first learn the meaning of the most indispensable words in order to understand what is said to us in the foreign tongue.

Till the beginning of this century very confused notions prevailed as to the activity of the brain and spinal cord. Luigi Rolando, the celebrated physiologist of the University of Turin, was the first who clearly showed that the medulla oblongata (that part of the spinal cord which lies nearest the brain) must be regarded as the centre of the whole nervous system. No one in his time knew the structure of the nerve-centres better than he, and it was he who proved that the medulla oblongata 'is the first rudiment of the nervous system, the seat of physical sensibility, of instinct, the director

---

[6] Fontana: *Veleno della Vipera*, i. p. 317.

of voluntary movements, the centre of life, and the wonderful cause of most surprising phenomena known under the names of sympathies and consents.[7]

If one cuts the head of a duck off at a blow, it does not remain motionless but moves, flaps its wings and flutters along, as though it meant to make its escape. It is said that the Emperor Commodus caused the heads of the ostriches in the circus to be shot off with curved arrows, and that the birds still ran on till they reached the goal. If we cut the head of a dog off with a hatchet, we see that the trunk wags the tail. There is a curious irony in the fact, but it need not shock us, for the animal no longer feels. If an irritant is applied to the skin, it draws its tail between its legs as though it were afraid, although it is headless.

V

A difficult question confronts us here. There are some physiologists who maintain that the maid is blind, and that she performs her work without knowing what she does; that she pulls the cord when the bell rings, heats the stoves, cooks, cleans the utensils, sweeps the house, gives the rubbish to the dustman, and so on—but all this without power of discernment, acting like an automaton, unable to make the slightest change in what she does merely from habit. Others, again, maintain that she does possess a few fragments of intelligence, that at certain times she reasons too, and that the soul of the house does not dwell in the master alone.

It is a very difficult question; because, if it can be proved that the maid is blind and does everything from habit, one may also say that the master—poor man!—does not see much either, and that he has certainly not been able to teach the maid anything.

I say the question is difficult also because the names of the greatest living physiologists are connected with it. Goltz and Foster took a frog, destroyed its brain, and then plunged it into a vessel full of water. If the frog were then touched it might be seen, like other frogs in similar circumstances, to respond by swimming about and even jumping out of the vessel. The water was then warmed up to 40°. The frog remained motionless, nor did it feel that the water was growing hot; it did not try to leap out, and thus allowed the heat to increase until it was boiled without making any movement which might indicate sensation. Therefore the spinal cord alone cannot think. The frog moves like a machine whenever it feels those stimuli to which it is accustomed (like an automaton of which one must press a certain knob in order to produce a particular movement); it is indifferent to everything else, allowing itself to be burnt and boiled and never moving, because no pain is felt.

My friend Tiegel, professor of physiology in Japan, made another experiment. He took a snake and severed the head at a blow. While the trunk was writhing on the

---

[7] L. Rolando, *Saggio sopra la vera struttura del cervello e sopra le funzioni del sistema nervoso*, Sec. III. p. 140. Turin, 1828.

ground he touched it with a red-hot iron bar, and the snake wound itself round it and did not desist, although its flesh was burnt and skin charred. And so, in this case too, the spinal cord producing these movements is unreasoning.

But how to explain all the other apparently reasoning acts?

The structure of the nerve-centres can itself give an appearance of intelligence to results which are purely mechanical. Let us assume that the nerve-paths passing to the various muscles from one side or the other transmit more or less easily the stimuli given off from the spinal cord. A drop of vinegar having been put on the leg of a frog, as before mentioned, certain muscles will at once move—that is, those of which the nerves oppose the least resistance to the stimuli produced in the centre. But if the animal cannot remove the cause of the irritation, the latter accumulates in the spinal cord, so increasing in force that the nervous tension makes a way for itself along more resisting paths, thus giving rise to other less usual movements.

VI

During my medical career I had more than once an opportunity of seeing the human spinal cord injured or severed. The most interesting case was that of a peasant, who, in falling from a tree, had severed the spinal cord in the dorsal region a little below the shoulder-blades, with a pruning hook. He moved his arms, spoke, but did not feel the lower part of his body any longer, nor the pain which a wound he had on the shin-bone would otherwise have caused him, although the leg moved whenever we touched the sore in order to treat it.

Marshall Hall proved that all generative acts are dependent on the lower part of the spinal cord, and Brachet tells of a soldier who became the father of two children although the lower half of his body was paralysed and quite without feeling. The only thing we do not find in an animal with the spinal cord severed are those irregular movements of the part separated from the brain, corresponding by their spontaneity to those we call voluntary.

Frogs and other animals of which one has cut the spinal cord are in general motionless and paralysed in the parts separated from the brain; we must touch them in order to make them move. If one pinches or slightly presses the hind-paw of a dog with the spinal cord severed in the dorsal region, he moves it or draws it away, but does it unconsciously, as we do if we are touched while asleep. If the stimulus is strong, he moves the other leg and his tail; if stronger still, he moves his whole body and trembles.

Even when the brain is wanting, slight stimuli produce a wagging of the tail; strong stimuli the drawing of the tail between the legs. This proves that certain characteristic phenomena of fear are produced without any participation of the will or consciousness.

The liveliness and restlessness so characteristic of youth arise from the greater excitability of the nervous system, which one always notices in young animals. The age, race, and bodily condition render very dissimilar the reflex movements by which animals deprived of their brain respond, even when they are excited in the same manner. The differences observable in character correspond to anatomical and functional differences of the nerve-centres.

As it is impossible to find two men having all parts of their brain or spinal cord exactly alike, we infer that these differences in the structure of the nerve apparatus materially influence other functional differences which seem to depend on causes of a higher order known under the generic name of *will*. What many call free-will is only a fatal necessity, an indissoluble chain of causes and effects, of physical and mechanical actions, of automatic and unconscious reactions in the living machine.

VII

In order to understand certain phenomena of fear, we must first study a few peculiarities presented by the excitable portions of the nervous system. If one stimulates the nerve running through the frog's leg by very slight electric currents which are incapable of producing a contraction of the muscles, the force of the current may be slowly and evenly increased without the leg moving or in any way responding. This experiment shows us that the motor nerves do not respond to the stimulus as such, because the latter may be very strong without producing any visible effect, but that it is the rapid variations and changes which cause the convulsive movements.

Any pain or fear assailing us unexpectedly causes a great disturbance in the organism, but have a less serious effect when slowly developed.

There is always a more energetic response during the first moments of a sensation. This fact is true of all phenomena of the nervous system, and it is therefore unnecessary to give examples of what everyone knows from experience. This depends also upon the fact that the nervous system discharges a part of its energy at every reaction, so that when the animal is very weak it responds no more after the first two or three times.

We now understand why slight, unexpected emotions produce such intense perturbations in the organism, while very serious events for which we are prepared have in proportion much less effect.

VIII

Pliny, in speaking of fear making one close the eyes, relates that amongst twenty gladiators scarcely two were found who did not wink when suddenly menaced.[8]

---

[8] Plinius: *Historia naturalis*, lib. xi., p. 480.

It is striking that such slight causes produce movements so pronounced that we are not capable of suppressing them. We know that our friend will certainly not poke his finger into our eye, but the conviction that it is a joke does not suffice. Even if a thick pane of glass were between us and the approaching hand, with all the force of reason and will, many would be unable to avoid shutting the eyes, as though there were in us two natures: one, animal and unreasoning which commands, and the other human and intelligent which succumbs.

Again, when a gnat or a grain of dust gets into our eye, the eye closes irresistibly by an automatic mechanism quite independent of our will. Sometimes there is not only one contraction, but a somewhat complicated series of movements excited in parts distant from the stimulus.

As a convincing example, I shall communicate what I observed in an investigation of deglutition. This act, performed unceasingly during eating, is by no means voluntary, for if we try to repeat it a few times in succession we notice at once that, as soon as we have no saliva in the mouth, every effort to swallow is in vain. In order to swallow it is necessary that a morsel of food or some fluid should touch the mucous membrane of the posterior portion of the mouth. The sensory nerves stimulated in this way communicate to the spinal cord that a body is at the entrance of the œsophagus which must be sent to the stomach. Immediately a succession of orders is issued, one after the other, by the spinal cord, so that first the upper part of the œsophagus contracts and propels the morsel a short way down, then a further order causes a contraction of the next part, then comes another order whereupon a part still lower down contracts, and so all the successive portions of the œsophagus transmit the morsel one to another by means of various separate orders until it reaches the stomach.

We have, therefore, in our nervous system mechanisms which work automatically, and produce a series of contractions directed to one object, which may, at first sight, appear voluntary, but is, in reality, mechanical and unconscious. Some of these mechanisms we bring into the world with us. If one puts a finger into the mouth of a new-born child it begins to suck. It is a machine working without discernment, as if one had touched the spring of an automatic doll; no one teaches the child, he need not learn it at all in fact, for the fœtus in the womb makes exactly the same movement. So it is with the chicken, which pecks when just escaped from the shell. In this case, what gives rise to the movement is no longer immediate contact as that of the finger in the mouth, but the impression of light and sight, which indeed is nothing else but contact with distant things by means of the rays of light. Scarcely has the image of the grain formed itself in the eye of the chicken but it pecks at it.

It suffices to observe our movements with a little attention, in order to be convinced that a greater number of them are automatic than one thinks. When we step out of bed in winter and thrust our naked feet into our slippers, the foot has scarcely touched the cold leather but it withdraws, and an effort is necessary in order to resist. We notice, too, that when the shoemaker measures us for a pair of shoes, it is somewhat difficult to keep our foot still even though he does not tickle us. When one touches iron, a cup, or any other object which is very hot, the hand lets go at once. This is a very useful circumstance, because we often let go of a thing which might injure us before we have even become aware that it burns or pricks. And when we have lost consciousness through illness or any accident, the body takes care of itself, as during sleep, by automatically removing itself from anything which pricks, burns, chills, stings, or presses, and so on. If the pain produced by burning is faint, only the one side of the body moves, if it spreads and grows stronger, it affects the opposite side also, and in the highest degrees, the whole body.

This law, which was established by Pflüger, holds good for normal and uninjured animals as well as for those from which the brain has been removed and which are unconscious. It shows us that the postures and movements of the body, so characteristic of a man responding to sudden pain, do not depend on his will. All that is most characteristic in the phenomena of fear: the palpitation, shortness of breath, pallor, screams, flight, trembling, are reflex movements. The more physiology advances, the more the domain of free-will is restricted, and the greater the increase of involuntary movements.

CHAPTER III

THE BRAIN

I

An animal deprived of the brain is a machine which requires external stimuli in order to move. An uninjured animal is also a machine, but it differs from the other by that power in itself which renders it capable of moving and acting.

When an animal with its brain removed is touched on any point of its body quite lightly, it does not respond at once to this external stimulus, and only when these light touches are often repeated is a reactionary movement excited. There are some very wonderful experiments which made a great impression on me, when I first saw them performed by my friends Kronecker and Stirling in the laboratory in Leipzig. They took a decapitated frog, and fastened between the toes of one of the hind-legs a pen, which made marks on the paper of a rotating cylinder whenever the frog moved. Between the toes of the other leg they fastened the wires of an electric current; a pendulum alternately opening and closing the current in such a manner that an interrupted stimulus was obtained. It was strange to see how the headless frog responded regularly for hours. When stimulated by a weak current (so weak that it could not be felt on the tongue) more numerous repetitions, perhaps thirty, were necessary before the frog responded by a spasmodic movement. If the stimulus were stronger a much smaller number was sufficient to cause reaction, and this continued until life was extinct.

Stimuli accumulate in the spinal cord. We all know it from experience; when we have something in the throat which tickles us, the slight, and at first scarcely perceptible, irritation becomes almost unbearable if it continues, compelling us to cough in order to remove it. As the Italian proverb says, one cannot disguise a cough. Even a slight tickling of the skin has the same effect, and in the functions of reproduction the repetition of slight stimuli produce greater and more ungovernable reflex movements.

There are, however, impressions which remain longer accumulated in the brain before their energy finds expression in muscular activity. Sometimes a part of the nervous system charges itself slowly, like a Leyden jar under the influence of weak electric sparks, the tension of the nerve-cells remaining, as it were, hidden, until suddenly discharged by a contact or some very slight impression. We are astonished; it seems an accidental explosion to us, an effect out of all proportion to the momentary cause, forgetting that fire glows under ashes, that the force had been slowly accumulating, and so we believe we have accomplished the act by means of the will.

The aptitude of the nerve-cells to accumulate and preserve external impressions is such a leading fact in physiology that I do not know any more important one.

If I were asked the difference between the brain and the spinal cord, I should say that the brain is more capable of accumulating impressions, not because of the difference of its substance, but because in it the nerve-cells serving this purpose are found in greater abundance.

The manner in which the brain has formed itself in the evolution of the animal world will render the comprehension of its activities easier. Let us consider the simplest creatures, those possessing, so to speak, only a spinal cord. The nerves branching off from the upper part to the nostrils, eyes, ears, mouth, and elsewhere, were subjected during the long series of generations to more continuous stimuli than other nerves. The cells placed at the roots of these nerves were constantly excited by impressions from the external world; chemical processes and combustion would be more rapid in them, hence the necessity of a more copious flow of blood to those parts which were in greater activity. These cells multiplied rapidly at the roots of the organs of sense, gradually covering a wider field. As the animal structure became more perfect during evolution, and the relations of the animal to the outer world increased, the more abundant and active the cells at the roots of these nerves would become. We must not think here of one individual, although individual exercise does strengthen an organ, but must fix our eyes on the interminable chain of generations, all working in this direction.

It was heredity (by which we still transmit to our children the structure and functions acquired by the nerve-centres) which, through the incessant efforts of our progenitors, enlarged this fertile field, until at last it resulted in the mass of the brain.

If, on visiting a museum of comparative anatomy, the reader will look into the glass cases set apart for the study of the nervous system, he will see that the lowest animals have only a spinal cord, or a very small protuberance at the place corresponding to the brain. As the animal structure becomes more complicated, there is a visible increase of the protuberance, which enlarges gradually the nearer one approaches the superior animals, until at last it reaches its maximum size in man.

II

One of the greatest experimenters of modern physiology, Flourens, had already given it as his opinion that the whole cerebral mass performs the same functions in all its parts, and that if one portion be taken away, those contiguous to it charge themselves with its offices. This affords a partial explanation of the fact that wounds of the brain are far less dangerous than those of the spinal cord. It is always a great wonder, even to us physiologists, every time we convince ourselves on living subjects that the brain is without feeling. Men have been seen who suffered great portions of their brain, which protruded from the skull, to be cut away, and sick drunkards or madmen, who, through the wounds in their head, seized hold of the brain with their hands and destroyed it.

Only in the last few years have physiologists succeeded in preserving alive for some time dogs of which nearly all the convolutions of the brain had been removed. Professor Goltz brought a dog in this state from Strasburg to London, in order to show the phenomena which an animal then presents, at the International Congress of Medicine. I extract a few fragments from Professor Goltz's work,[9] in order to give an idea of the phenomena exhibited by dogs when deprived of a great part of their brain.

A brainless dog has a stupid, inane look. One reads idiocy even in his eyes. His movements are slow and uncertain. It seems as though he needed far more time than usual to come to a decision. His gait is like that of a goose, there is something inexpressibly strange and comical in it. The animal always walks straight on like an automaton. If he meets another dog, he steps over him if he is little; if he is big he may lift him with his head, or knock him down, but on he goes. He tries awkwardly to step over every object he meets, although by simply stepping aside he might pass on without hindrance. He only finds his dish of food with difficulty, smell guiding him better than sight; he snaps stupidly at everything he sees, even biting his own paws till he howls with pain. He can no longer find the fragments of bone that fall out of his mouth while chewing.

Dogs like these are no longer capable of learning anything, and one might almost say that they have forgotten what they already knew; for instance, they no longer give their paw to their master, as they used to do. Their whole intellectual life is extinguished; only when they hear a knock at the door do they bark, but they always begin too late. Two dogs that hated each other, bit each other when they met, even after both had lost a great part of their brain. Memory diminishes in proportion as larger quantities of the brain are removed, and disappears wholly when nearly the whole organ is wanting.

III

In order better to understand the working of the brain, we may divide it in imagination into two parts: a lower, situated at the base of the cerebral hemispheres, which forms the direct continuation of the spinal cord and is the centre of those movements which arise involuntarily during emotion; and another part in the upper story, as it were, which consists of the cerebral convolutions, is also in connection with the spinal cord, and must be considered as the seat of voluntary movement.

The enormous difference between the mind of a man and that of a child exists because in the latter the upper story of the brain is not developed, the convolutions are scarcely indicated, the organs of will and speech are wanting. As the large pyramidal cells appear and increase, the child acquires intelligence and speech; connections are

---

[9] F. Goltz: *Ueber die Verrichtungen des Grosshirns*, p. 61, and following. Bonn, 1881.

established with the lower story in order to set muscles and organs which were before inactive into movement. But the difference between these two stories of nerve-centres continues during the whole life. I shall explain this by a few examples. A man is paralysed in consequence of some injury which prevents the upper story of his brain from communicating with the spinal cord. Hands and arms no longer move under the influence of the will, but when some long-expected person appears, or some sudden shock is given to the emotional sphere, he will be able to lift his arms. There is a paralysis of the facial nerve in which the voluntary closing of the eye is impossible, but if anyone makes a movement, as though he were going to poke his finger into the eye, the lid closes instantly. Later, we shall instance men who have remained dumb for a long time, and have regained their speech in consequence of a fright.

Dogs deprived of a large part of the upper story of the brain make no sign of recognition when they see themselves threatened by the whip, but if it is cracked they scamper off hurriedly, or rush forward at it. A mouse with its hemispheres and optic thalami removed remained undisturbed by every noise but that resembling an approaching cat, when it jumped and fled.

By means of injuries to the brain physiologists can easily check the activity of certain voluntary movements. If the peduncles of the cerebellum and certain points of the cerebrum are injured, dogs can be made to go either only to the right, or to the left, continually backwards, or in a circle, as though they were in a circus. The will of the animal is still in existence, but all his efforts are, as often with us, fruitless. In spite of himself his body is drawn in the direction determined by the lesion of the nerve-centres. Claude Bernard tells of a brave old general who, by a cruel irony of fate, could only march backwards.

Many physiologists have of late years tried to establish with precision the point of the brain which is the seat of emotional expressions; that is, that part, the destruction of which obliterates every expression of fear or pain in the animal, although allowing life to continue. One of the latest works published concerning this is by Bechterew. His observations show that a dog, in whose brain the corpora bigemina and quadrigemina have been destroyed, still barks and shows his teeth if anything loathsome is given him to eat, or if something smelling disagreeably is put before him; but that he is bereft of all expression of disgust and loathing after the two optic thalami have been removed. Hence Bechterew concludes that the paths of transmission along which pass the involuntary commands which cause the muscles to contract, in order to express the emotions, concentrate in the optic thalamus, which is one of the deepest parts of the brain. The upper story of volition and the lower of the emotions have here their point of union, whence to excite in the muscles of the organism all the characteristic movements of the passions.

IV

Let us now see what instinctive qualities we inherit from our forefathers, and what others we acquire through our own experience.

Long ago Galen performed a very simple and instructive experiment. He cut a kid out of the body of its mother, laid it immediately on the ground, and, near its head, dishes in which were oil, wine, honey, vinegar, water, and milk. He then stood to observe the first movements of the animal. After trembling a little, the kid got up, scratched itself, smelt a few of the dishes, and at last drank the milk.

There are birds which, scarcely out of the shell, catch flies with such precision that one is astonished at their bringing with them skill such as must usually be acquired by long practice. Certain butterflies, on leaving the cocoon, fly at once into the air, directing their flight with the most perfect accuracy towards the flowers, to suck the nectar from their cups.

We shall return to this point when we investigate fear in children. Let us here only state that, at his birth, man is far less perfect than many animals. He must acquire by education and experience much knowledge of which animals are possessed at the beginning.

The less care parents give to their young, the more completely do they furnish them through heredity with instinctive knowledge; the less considerable this inheritance, the more care and attention must parents give to their offspring in order to keep them alive.

This apparent inferiority in the gifts of instinct at birth is, as it is with the gifts of fortune, fully compensated for by the greater capability of those animals to increase their intellectual capacity by education, and by the work of their own experience to surpass by far animals more favoured by instinct; so it is with man, who subjugates them all.

Let us think of the tremendous difficulties which walking presents to man. Children are at first very much afraid of falling, even before they have experienced such a thing. Every movement is performed with difficulty; it is at first a task painfully learnt; gradually it becomes less a matter of reflection, until at last one can scarcely call it voluntary. We may not call it automatic, because when the will to make us walk is wanting we do not move, but when we have once set out on a walk, or to make a journey, we may go on for a long time without reflecting in the least that we are walking.

Ribot[10] tells of a violoncellist who suffered from epileptic vertigo, during which he became unconscious. He earned his living by playing in the orchestra of a theatre, and it was often noticed that he continued playing in time, even after he had lost consciousness. It has happened to all of us to read aloud without understanding what

---

[10] Th. Ribot: *Les Maladies de la Mémoire*, p. 9. Paris, 1881.

we have read, or absent-mindedly to write one word for another, and many will have experienced such extreme fatigue that they have slept while walking. There are endless phenomena proving that movements which at first cost a great effort of the will, become at length so habitual that we perform them without being aware of it.

Now what is the cause of this transformation of voluntary into automatic movements?

When we first try to execute a series of complicated movements the brain must work hard. If the cells of the upper story—that is, of the convolutions—do not take part in it, it all comes to nothing; the assistance of all the organs of sense is necessary in order to shed light on the confusion of orders and counter orders which must be sent to all the fibres of the muscles. The work is accomplished under the direction of a competent, enlightened administration; but through repetition of the same work, easier paths, broader lines of communication are formed in the lower story of the brain, and gradually the same work can be performed by the cells of the lower part— that is, without the co-operation of the will. This is easy to understand. The oftener a thing is repeated, the more the mechanism tends to become permanent, and it ends in the work being despatched by the less noble parts of the brain.

The serious aspect of the question is, that physiologists would like to catalogue many qualities which we have always considered as the most noble of our character, the most sublime feelings of human nature, amongst the automatic movements and more material instincts in the lower story of the brain.

For instance, for the maintenance of our species the love of the mother for her children is indispensable. The lower animals that produce a numerous offspring may carelessly abandon them, but when the progeny is sparse, there is no other way to preserve the species than through the greater and more prolonged attention on the part of the parents.

Let us for a moment study the character of the monkey. I quote from the celebrated book by Brehm, who conscientiously relates what he himself noticed.

'When the monkey-suckling is unable to do anything for itself, the mother is all the more gentle and tender with it. She occupies herself with it unceasingly, sometimes licking it, sometimes running after it or embracing it, looking at it as though revelling in the sight of it; then she lays it against her breast and rocks it to sleep. When the little monkey grows bigger the mother grants him a little freedom, but she never loses sight of him; she follows his every step and does not permit him to do everything he likes. She washes him in the brooks and smooths his fur with loving care.

'At the least danger she rushes to him with a cry, warning him to take refuge in her arms. Any disobedience is punished with pinches or cuffs, but this seldom happens, for the monkey does not do what its mother objects to. The death of the young one is, in many cases, followed by that of the mother from grief.[11] After a fight monkeys generally leave their wounded on the field; only the mothers defend their young against every enemy, however formidable. At first the mother tries to escape with the young one, but if she falls, she emits a loud cry of pain and remains still, in a threatening attitude, with wide-open mouth, gnashing her teeth, and menacing the enemy with outstretched arms.'

Davancel tells of the profound emotion he experienced after having killed a monkey. 'The poor animal had a young one with her, and the bullet hit her in the region of the heart. She made a last effort, placed the young one on the branch of a tree and then fell down dead. I have never felt,' he says, 'greater remorse at having killed a creature, which, even in dying, showed feeling so worthy of admiration.'[12]

Whether this is instinct or affection, whether there is any difference between the love of man and of the monkey, I do not feel called upon to decide. I acknowledge that it is necessary for the maintenance of the species that things should be thus, nor need our admiration for mechanisms made in this way suffer any diminution.

I do not think I deserve praise for loving my mother. I remember what she did for me; and even if all our affection were only a simple automatic correspondence of instincts, if I knew that neither had the power to act otherwise, I should be just as glad to be constituted in such a manner that I cannot repress the throbbings of my heart whenever her face rises in my memory. I do not think that my tears and sorrow show less of love on that account.

And if I still feel myself drawn to the grave of the mother who died long years ago, thus cherishing her memory by visiting it in the greatest joys and sorrows of my life, I am glad to be an automaton feeling the religion of love in this renewal of the grief and tears of the last farewell.

---

[11] Brehm: *Thierleben*, p. 49. Leipzig, 1883.

[12] Brehm: *Thierleben*, p. 106. Leipzig, 1883.

CHAPTER IV

THE CIRCULATION OF THE BLOOD IN THE BRAIN DURING EMOTION

I

When we have drawn on a pair of very tight gloves, we feel, if we pay attention, a slight throbbing in the fingers, corresponding to the rhythm of the cardiac pulsations. This throbbing arises because, by every contraction of the heart, one hundred and eighty cubic centimetres of blood—that is, about as much as can be contained in an ordinary drinking-glass—are driven out of the cavity of the thorax. As this wave of blood penetrates the various organs of the body they swell, as is the case with the arteries which dilate at every pulsation and then resume their former volume. When the hands are unconfined we notice nothing, but if we squeeze them into gloves, or our feet into tight shoes, we feel something beating in fingers and toes. This is the blood gushing in, and as the skin cannot yield as in ordinary conditions, the extremely delicate nerve-filaments which branch into it are pressed at every pulsation. If our finger swells from a whitlow, an inflammation, a knock or a burn, immediately the physiological pulsations, unnoticed before, become continuous, causing an acute, stinging pain. The blood flows more abundantly to the inflamed part, the elasticity of the tissues diminishes, the skin becomes more unyielding, an increased pressure on the nerves ensues, and these, rendered more sensitive through the injury, communicate a painful sensation to the brain which pricks unceasingly, keeping time with the rhythm of the heart.

In no organ is the supply of blood so abundant as in the brain; it is sufficient to state that one-fifth of the blood in our body goes to the head. Often, when lying on our side with our cheek on the pillow, we hear the waves of blood passing from the heart to the brain. The arteries, in pulsating, raise the skin, and this movement occasions a slight friction against the pillow, which then propagates itself to the ear. But it is not the beating of the blood against the walls of the vessels, as we feel it on the carotid artery of the neck, or on the radial artery of the hand and elsewhere, which most interests us. A whole world of important facts in the physiology of the emotions and in the circulation of the blood would still be unknown if physicians were still only feeling the pulse, as has been done from the earliest days of medicine until now.

With the old methods we should never have succeeded in observing the spectacle of continuous and ever-varying changes which the movement of the blood operates in the brain, the hand, or the foot.

The physiologist used to be like a man wishful to study the life of a city, and only able to do this by looking down from a terrace at the coming and going of the crowd, the perpetual stream of people in the street. Only of late years have we succeeded in penetrating into the houses by the roof, in spying out the inner life of each family, in studying the irrigation of the organs by the blood while they are at work or in repose.

The pulse in the finest branches of the vessels and in the inward recesses of the organs is such a subtile, delicate phenomenon that we need the assistance of special instruments to intensify it before we can study it. I shall not do as many naturalists do, who think they should conceal the artistic side of their investigations from the fear of desecrating science.

I know that every experimental work possesses an interesting side, which is quite lost owing to the aridity and severity with which scientific treatises are written, and I therefore abandon myself to the recollections of my investigations, careless of following the style of popular scientific books.

II

The first work which I published upon the circulation of blood in the human brain brings sad recollections to me. It was in June 1875 that my friend, Professor Carlo Giacomini, invited me to visit one of his patients in the syphilitic ward. It was a peasant woman, thirty-seven years of age, who, after having borne six children, had been infected by her husband with the most terrible disease to which a mother may fall a victim. For nine years the deadly poison had raged in her bones, and, with only short intervals of respite, had corroded a great part of the skeleton and destroyed the upper part of the skull from the nasal bones to the occiput. Medical art had proved powerless to arrest the disease. When Professor Giacomini took the woman out of pity into the hospital, her face was disfigured, her body was covered with sores and scars, the skin of the head was detached in various parts, the corroded skull had a blackish colour, like dead bones encased in living flesh.

It was after hearing from this unhappy woman the story of her misfortune, and during the intense emotion which pity for her aroused, that I saw for the first time, through the fissures of the decayed bones, the movement of the uncovered brain. Even to-day, eight years later, when I think of that moment, a shiver runs over me as it did then.

The patient recovered strength after energetic treatment, and was able to walk about the garden after a few weeks. It was then that we began to study her brain. I shall not describe the various instruments we constructed, but only remark that we lost much precious time with different attempts, and when we were at last ready, the most favourable time was already past, the wound was covered with a thick scab, which dulled the pulse of the brain. Nevertheless, we made some rather important observations, the results obtained being the most complete up till that time in the physiology of cerebral circulation.

In order to give an instance of the delicacy of the apparatus, and to prove the accuracy of our investigations, I mention the following circumstance. One day we were assembled in the laboratory of Professor Giacomini, intent on studying the brain of the patient, who was sitting in her arm-chair, and seemed absent-minded. There were a few spectators in the room, who were told to remain quietly behind the patient's back. In solemn silence we observed the curve marked by the cerebral pulse on the registering apparatus. Suddenly, without any external cause, the pulsations rose higher, and the brain increased in size. This striking me as strange, I asked the woman how she felt; the answer was, well. Seeing, however, that the circulation in the brain was very much altered, I examined the instrument carefully, to see whether it was all in order. Then I asked the patient to tell me most minutely what she had been thinking about two minutes before. She said that, as she had been looking absent-mindedly into a bookcase standing opposite to her, she had caught sight of a skull between the books, adding that it had frightened her by reminding her of her malady.

This poor woman was called Margherita; she was rather timid, but willingly allowed herself to be examined and studied, full of confidence in us, who vied with each other in showing her polite attentions. Her children often visited her, but she was ashamed to go back to her native place with her terribly disfigured face, preferring to remain away from her family and perform the duties of nurse to the other invalids in the hospital. After many years I felt a wish to see her again. As I pressed her hand to encourage her, she told me that she had at last given up the wish to die.

III

Chance furthered the continuation of these observations, new opportunities for this study soon offering themselves in Turin and elsewhere. In the lunatic asylum I found a boy a portion of whose skull was wanting. In the year 1877 I came across a man in the hospital of San Giovanni, who had an opening in his forehead which seemed made on purpose for examination; and finally, last year, I was able to repeat and conclude my investigations on a perfectly healthy man who had also a hole in his skull. As yet I have had no opportunity of publishing the observations and experiments made on this man.

How anxious and agitated we are when we enter upon a new field of science; when, at every step, the doubt arises whether some important phenomenon may not have escaped us! How we are tormented by the fear of not being able to face the most vital questions, nor to find out those phenomena most fruitful in results and most subtle! What trepidation overcomes one before one writes down even a few lines in the book of science!

Even amongst physicians it is not easy to find any who are able to write down the history of any fact or observation. The majority of them only know how to relate things in the same dogmatic words with which they are described in treatises, and only a few take the trouble to examine the development of an idea. And yet, in the study of human nature there is nothing more interesting than to follow the different phases of a problem, to see whence a thought arose, to know the first means by which nature was interrogated, then the sudden changes of method, the incidents, the errors and corrections, and at last the victory which crowns our labour and wins a fact for science. I believe if it could be seen near at hand how a research develops in the laboratories, the followers of the experimental sciences would be greater in number.

It is a work of patience. The only difficulty consists in gradually learning the language of Nature, in finding out the way to interrogate her and compel her to reply. In this struggle, in which we, humble pygmies, fight continually in order to wrest from Life its secret, there are moments of intoxicating emotion, rays of light amongst the shadows, which excite the imagination of the scholar and the artist.

IV

The second case, which I studied in company with Dr. Albertotti, was that of a boy eleven years of age, with an agreeable physiognomy and very beautiful physical proportions. He had scarcely reached his second year when he fell from a terrace, fracturing his skull and causing a severe concussion of the brain. After two years and a half he began to suffer from epileptic fits, and later, signs of insanity appeared which obliged his relatives to send him to the lunatic asylum in Turin.

When I saw him in February 1877, he had a large opening in the skull, a little above the right eye, and covered with skin; it was as big as the palm of his hand, and in the pit of it one could feel the pulsing of the brain. The terrible fall had for ever arrested his intellectual development. He was gay, smiling, and lively, like a big baby, but he could not speak. It was a saddening circumstance that in the midst of this ruin of his mind one single higher idea had remained, a remnant of his earlier intellectual life, a motto which he constantly repeated: 'I want to go to school.'

Of all the human cases I have studied, the observations made on this boy gave me the greatest trouble. As I had to do with an idiot, the least obstacles became great difficulties. No apparatus could be applied without his becoming restless, snatching it from his head, and breaking everything which fell into his hands. I had to confine myself to a few observations which could be made by surprising him while asleep. But he did not sleep regularly; I have often found him still awake, even when I made my nightly visit at a very late hour. It was more than sleeplessness, it was a nocturnal excitement, which presaged the storm of an epileptic attack. I have seen him the victim of the most terrible fits, while, on the nights following, his sleep was so deep as to leave one in doubt whether it was a natural phenomenon.

In the period of exhaustion and stupor, the blood-vessels of the brain seemed to relax, and at every contraction of the heart the pulsations became stronger. A faint noise which did not wake the patient was enough to produce a change in the brain and a more abundant gush of blood. It sufficed to touch him, or to approach him with the lamp: immediately, the volume of the brain increased, and a great elevation appeared in the curve of the pulse.

Whenever we called him by name, it seemed as though an impetuous wave of blood rushed into the brain, causing the convolutions to swell. As this was invariably the case, there could be no doubt that the brain was still sensitive to the impressions of the external world, even during a heavy sleep. When the patient was shaken till he woke, I could see the circulation changing little by little, as though the material conditions of consciousness were being restored.

He often spoke a few indistinct words, opened his eyes, or moved his hands, and then slowly fell back into the previous stupor, while we saw the pulse grow weaker, the brain decrease in volume, the rhythm and force of the breathing change.

It was one of the most interesting sights to observe in the stillness of night, by the light of a little lamp, what was going on in his brain, when there was no external cause to disturb this mysterious life of sleep. The brain-pulse remained for ten or twenty minutes quite regular and very weak, and then began suddenly, without any apparent cause, to swell and beat more vigorously. Then the agitation subsided and there was a second period of quiet; then came stronger blood-waves which flooded the convolutions, raising the height of the pulsations, which were automatically marked by the apparatus applied to the brain. We scarcely dared breathe. The one who was observing the instruments communicated with the other, who was watching over the patient, by pressing his hand. Looks full of interrogation and wonder would meet, and exclamations had to be forcibly repressed.

Did dreams, perhaps, come to cheer the repose of the unhappy boy? Did the face of his mother and the recollections of his early childhood grow bright in his memory, lighting up the darkness of his intelligence and making his brain pulsate with excitement? Or was it perhaps only a morbid phenomenon, like the jerky movements of a broken wheel, or the index of a machine out of order, swinging idly to and fro? Or was it an unconscious agitation of matter, like the ebb and flow of an unknown and solitary sea?

What a contrast between the pleasing emotion which this work roused in us and the sadness of the surroundings! Even that quarter of the city in which the asylum is situated has something characteristic about it, which De Amicis compared to the silence and mystery of an Oriental town. Sometimes, when late on winter evenings I made my way along the deserted streets, I could not even hear my own footsteps as they fell noiselessly on the snow. In the long dormitories of the hospital the dim light of the lamp could not dissipate the gloom in the remote corners of the room. However much care I took to glide softly through the room, in order not to disturb the sleep of those poor wretches, many were yet sitting upright in their beds, with staring eyes, seeming to await my coming and ready to shriek at me as I passed. Others, uncovered and naked, in spite of the winter cold, gazed at me with empty, fixed eyes; while others again, bound, to prevent their injuring either themselves or others in their mad fury, followed my steps with wild glances.

What a cheerless sight for a physician, and for me, who came amongst them to study the brain. At the end of these rooms was a little chamber in which I watched my subject. Often I had to interrupt my investigations, and, lamp in hand, go to the most noisy, begging, imploring them to be silent for one minute. It was a waste of breath. Caresses, presents, threats—all were alike of no avail. And when, late at night, discouraged at the failure of my experiments, I left that abode of pain, they were still awake, staring at me with the fixed, impenetrable gaze of a sphynx or the malignant smile of a demon; and when I stepped out into the desolate street again it seemed to me as though I had just escaped from a vision of spectres.

V

Physiologists may wait a long time before finding a more suitable subject on which to study the circulation of blood in the brain than my Bertino. He had a hole in the very middle of the forehead, that seemed made to allow one to look into the skull as an old Greek philosopher once wished to do with the human heart.

To my regret the man only sojourned for a very short time in Turin, and I could only study him during one week. He was a sturdy mountaineer, who suffered from home-sickness, and seemed to be ashamed of his disfigurement. In July 1877, as he was working under the belfry of his village, he was struck on the head by a brick which a mason, working near the roof, at a height of fourteen metres, let fall out of his hand. Bertino fell to the ground as though struck by lightning. He told me that he remembered nothing of it all, not even the blow he had received, and that he regained consciousness after one hour. The earliest recollection which he preserved of the accident was of the moment before the blow. He remembered that he was standing under the belfry watching a comrade dipping bricks into water; then came a period of darkness in his mind, and when he came to himself again he found himself, to his astonishment, in bed, while a surgeon held a watch before him and asked him what time it was. From that moment his mind had been quite clear. The terrible blow made an opening of the size of a shilling in the middle of the forehead. When the splinters of bone had been removed, the brain was seen through the opening, uncovered and pulsating. After having been twenty-four hours in bed, he came on foot to Turin. My friend, Dr. De Paoli, took me to see him. The patient had lost nothing of his power of movement, of his intelligence, his speech, or his memory; he was only very much afraid, and had a perpetual expression of distrust and timidity, even about the most unimportant things, which he tried in vain to conceal.

I must remark that in fractures of the skull the time favourable to study is very short. Large wounds admit with difficulty of the application of the instruments; the smaller ones are better adapted, but they close much sooner from underneath by cicatrisation. When I made the acquaintance of Bertino, the best time was already past; nevertheless the investigations which I made on him are, according to the judgment of competent physiologists, the most complete that have as yet been published.

Eighteen months later I wrote to him, asking him to come to Turin, as I wished to see him. He came at once, and told me that if he had not escaped from the hospital he would have died of melancholy; that he had not been able to bear being in rooms full of dying people, while at home wife and children and fields were awaiting him. The opening in the skull had closed, and the movements of the brain were no longer visible.

VI

Let us now see how the brain writes when it guides the pen itself. I have already collected a few volumes of these autographs, from which I here give a single line as an example, written by Bertino's brain in the night of September 27, 1877. He was lying on a sofa. I had applied the apparatus which traces the movements of the brain to his forehead, and watched the pen writing on the cylinder while I waited for him to fall asleep. At first the pen traced large undulations, a certain sign of great restlessness in the blood-vessels of the brain; the pulse-lines were considerably modified from time to time in form and height, and this, although profound silence reigned. I might have asked him what he was thinking of, but I did not do it, as I wished urgently to see him fall asleep. At last the undulations began to decrease, becoming lower and less frequent, sometimes separated from each other by long periods of repose, like a lake gradually growing calm, but upon which from time to time a little wave ripples, troubling the smooth surface. At length Bertino fell asleep. Consciousness was extinguished, the troublous thoughts of life had ceased, only the last sentinels of the nervous system were still vigilant. At the slightest noise a wave of blood disturbed the surface of the brain. If the hospital clock struck the hour, or someone walked along the terrace, if I moved my chair, or wound up my watch, or if a patient coughed in the next room—everything, the slightest sound was accompanied by a marked alteration in the circulation of the brain, all immediately traced by the pen which the brain guided on the paper of my registering apparatus.

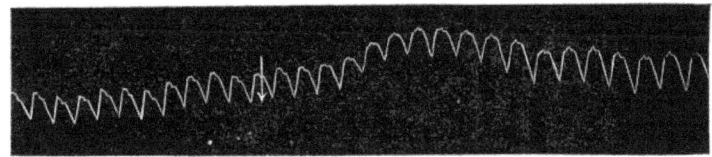

FIG. 1.—PULSE OF THE HUMAN BRAIN DURING SLEEP

After an hour and a half, when I saw that Bertino was breathing quite calmly, with the rhythm and in the characteristic manner of a sleeper, I rose with great caution, approached the pillow on which he had laid his head, and at that point in the curve where is the sign of the arrow, ↓, I called him gently by name, 'Bertino.' He did not move or answer. If we examine the curve in fig. 1, we find that even before the sign, ↓, four pulsations are somewhat higher than the preceding ones. This first increase in the volume of the brain is due to the very slight noise which I involuntarily made with the chair on rising to approach Bertino.

After calling him by name, the brain wrote three pulsations which have the form of the preceding ones; then the pulse changed, and the pen traced four pulsations, one higher than the other. This is the beginning of what I have called an *undulation*. During the next pulsations the pulse-line gradually falls until it reaches the previous height. In comparing the form of the pulsations at the beginning of this curve with those at the end, we see that even this very slight emotion, which was not able to interrupt sleep, yet sufficed to produce a great modification. The pulse is stronger, its form tricuspid. We physiologists would say that, from being anacrotic, it had become catacrotic. But the variations which appear in the circulation of the brain during fear are far greater. The reproofs and threats which I uttered to Bertino when he was hindering my experiments by moving his head or hands, the disagreeable things which I sometimes purposely said to him, were always followed by very strong pulsations; the brain-pulse became six, seven times higher than before, the blood-vessels dilated, the brain swelled and palpitated with such violence that physiologists were astonished when they saw the reproductions of the curves, published in the tables of my researches on the circulation of the brain.[13]

VII

In Canada, in 1822, a soldier called Alexis St. Martin was shot at from a short distance. The bullet penetrated the abdomen, perforating the stomach. In a few months, thanks to the treatment of Dr. Beaumont, he was completely healed, only an opening remained in the abdominal walls through which the processes in the stomach could be seen. Several physiologists in America had thus the opportunity of observing the stomach during digestion by looking into its cavity as through a window. The investigations made on this soldier resulted in the statement that the stomach becomes redder as soon as digestion begins. Later, physiologists showed, by other observations, that the salivary glands grow red during mastication, and that the muscles contain more blood when they are at work a long time. We all know that the eyes of anyone who works long become red, that the feet swell after a long walk, and that, in fencing, the muscles of the arms and the hand which grasp the weapon grow thicker.

From these facts we may deduce a law which has no exceptions, namely, that blood is more copiously supplied to an active organ.

The organs of our body are like so many little machines, to which one must furnish fuel if their working power is to be increased. But whereas, in ordinary mechanisms, it is a strange hand which keeps up the fire and directs the movements,

---

[13] *R. Accademia dei Lincei,* vol. v. series 3a; *Nuova Antologia,* March 1881.

our organism is so perfect that in it all apparatus regulate themselves with the greatest harmony of object. In the working muscle the blood-vessels expand, thus more easily to transmit the fuel, and in order that the muscle may convert the chemical force of food into a contraction. In the digesting stomach the circulation is more abundant, because the glands must secrete a greater quantity of juice, the little veins absorb the fluids contained in the stomach, and the muscles contract more quickly in order to mix the food.

Our organism, like all working machines, not only consumes and destroys fuel, here represented by those elements which constitute the blood, but through its activity it also wastes those parts of the body which represent the wheels, axles, hinges, and other parts of a mechanism. At every contraction of the muscles, at every sensation in the brain and nerves during any mental work, there is a wasting of the organs. The blood, flowing continually through all parts of the body in order to feed the flame of life, sweeps at the same time the most remote corners of our organism clean of soot, or the remains of combustion. The vessels become relaxed and expand. Nutrition and organic change become more rapid, the nutritive fluid trickles more easily through the walls of the vessels, the blood flows more quickly, and carries everywhere along with it all the waste products in order to bring them to the kidneys. These purify the blood, and expel, with the urine, the scoriæ of the working organism.

We have seen how the circulation in the brain is accelerated during mental activity, emotion, and in a waking condition; we shall return to this subject in the next chapter, and study more nearly the mechanism by which such variations are produced in all the other organs of the body. This subject is of great importance to physiologists, because in no other way can the slender link which connects psychological phenomena with the material functions of the organism be rendered more evident.

It suffices to increase or diminish in a slight degree the rapidity of the blood penetrating to the brain, in order to cause an immediate change of our 'ego.' The equilibrium of the molecules in the organs where consciousness has its seat is greatly disturbed by causes which scarcely affect the functions of other parts of the body; because, in the brain, nutrition is more active, and the state of the substances composing it more unstable. The sublimity of psychic phenomena has its root in the greater complication of the material facts by which they are originated. If I were asked which of the functions of the organism were most sensitive to the slightest organic change, I should, without hesitation, answer—*consciousness.*

VIII

Often, in contemplating the brain of my patients, pondering over its structure and functions, and seeing the blood coursing through it, I have imagined that I might penetrate into the inner life of the brain-cells, might follow the movements which agitate their minute branches in the labyrinth of the nerve-centres; I have thought I might learn the laws of organic change, the order, harmony, the most perfect concatenations; but my mind might work as it listed, and imagination seize the reins, I never yet saw anything, not the faintest gleam, which gave me hope of penetrating to the source of thought.

During my investigations I have discovered the mechanism with which nature provides for a more rapid circulation of blood when the brain must enter into activity; I was the first to admire some of the phenomena in which the material activity of this organ reveals itself; but although I have scrutinised the functions of the brain with the most exact methods of physiological investigation while it was pulsing under my eyes, while ideas were seething in it, or while it rested in sleep, the nature of the psychic processes still remains a mystery.

We all believe that the faculties of the mind are the fruit of an uninterrupted series of natural causes, of physical and chemical actions which lead from the simplest reflex-movements, step by step, to instinct, reason, sentiment, and will; but as yet nothing has been found which might lead us even to suspect, much less to comprehend, the nature of consciousness.

We attain our firmest convictions in the domain of positivism, not from the narrow field of physiology but from the whole kingdom of science. We imagine that the impressions of the external world form a current which penetrates the nerves, and, without either abatement or check, diffuses and transforms itself in the centres, finally reappearing in the sublime form of the idea; this is the notion of the soul held by the philosophers of remote antiquity; this is the base of modern psychology.

We may suppose that thought must be a form of motion, because the science of the present day demonstrates that all intimately known phenomena may be reduced to a vibration of atoms and to a displacement of molecules.

I can think of my brain by the analogy which it must have with that of another; but the bridge which leads me from external to internal observations I cannot find; between physical and psychic phenomena there is a gulf which we cannot pass.

The soul was regarded by the ancients as a harmony. But how this sublime harmony of imagination, of memory, of the passions, and of thought, results from the vibration of the molecules constituting the brain, no one knows. The road which connects psychic facts with the transformation of energy has not yet been pointed out.

I know the chemical transformations which give rise to the mechanical work of the muscles of my hand in writing, but I do not know the processes of my brain which thinks and dictates.

Many have thought and asserted, because the muscles and glands of our body grow heated by their work, that the brain and nerves also grew warm during activity. For my part, I doubt the accuracy of the methods used in these experiments, nor shall I be convinced unless it be clearly shown to be a fact. As the nature of the chemical processes taking place in the brain is totally unknown to us, it may be that the brain grows colder during activity. The question can only be decided when we succeed in eliminating the serious complications which the greater flow of blood produces in such cases.

Till the present day no one knows what parts of the brain are consumed in order to produce thought; no one can imagine how the molecules of the blood penetrate the mass of cerebral cells and become part of consciousness, and neither do we know how, from the joint life of the single cells, something can arise which represents consciousness and sensitivity.

Doctrines are here of no use. When our mind has arrived at the last division of matter, at the last localisation of psychic processes, we feel that it is vain to say we are materialists or spiritualists. All schools are confounded in the nullity of our ignorance. The nature of matter is as incomprehensible as that of spirit. From Lucretius, who gave thirty proofs to demonstrate the materiality of the soul, down to modern materialists, not one step has been taken towards the discovery of the nature of thought. As a matter of fact, many materialists throw down one dogma and build another out of its ruins.

If we reject the hypothesis of the spiritualists, we must, with the same severity, banish from the borders of experimental science those who, in our time, wish to explain, by means of materialistic doctrines, the mechanism generating thought. Anatomy and physiology, the knowledge of structure and of cerebral functions, have scarcely lisped their first words, and dense darkness reigns over the nature of nervous processes, over the physical and chemical movements animating the hidden parts where consciousness has its throne. Let us speak neither of spirit nor of matter; let us candidly acknowledge our ignorance. We trust to the future of science and persevere in the search after truth.

CHAPTER V

PALLOR AND BLUSHING

I

Man has, on the average, four kilograms of blood, and this fluid flows incessantly in a system of tubes, in the centre of which the heart is situated. The arteries carrying the blood from the heart to the surface divide into many branches, separate, extend, and visit all parts of the body, feeding and irrigating them. When the ramifications of the arteries become so small that the eye can no longer see them, as, for instance, in the lips, the finger-tips, the cheeks, the ears, or any part of the skin, they take the name of capillaries. This is meant to indicate that these little arteries are as fine as a hair, but in reality they are very much finer. These last closely connected capillary nets give the skin its beautiful rosy colour. But however much they diminish, dividing and subdividing *ad infinitum*, they still form a system of canals, with walls and closed on all sides. There must be a wound, a cut, or a contusion, before the blood oozes out of these little vessels. Out of the capillaries the blood passes into larger canals called veins. Several veins flowing into each other form a bigger vein; in the same way as a brook is formed by springs, as the brooks, running into each other, form a rivulet, and the rivulets, a river; so the veins gradually receive the blood in larger streams, until at last they carry it in the great trunk-veins to the heart, which drives it again into the arteries.

The little canals in which the blood circulates are provided with muscular fibre. These may relax and the calibre of the vessels is increased, or they contract and the calibre is reduced. The pallor, so characteristic of fear, arises from a contraction of the vessels; the beautiful blush of modesty, most eloquent of all the revelations of psychic facts, is nothing else but a dilatation of the blood-vessels. These two opposite phenomena do not depend on the heart, since we know that the heart beats more forcibly and rapidly during the emotion of modesty as well as during fright. From the nerve-centres innumerable filaments branch off which are distributed to all the ramifications of the blood-vessels. These are the so-called vaso-motor nerves, which, without our noticing it, act on the muscular fibre of the small arteries and veins, increasing or diminishing the calibre of the little canals in which the blood flows.

The effects of the passions are far more evident on the countenance, with its blushing and sudden pallor, than elsewhere, because in no other part of the body are the blood-vessels so sensitive as in the face. There are two reasons for this, firstly, the nerve-centres act more powerfully on these vessels; secondly, they are more delicate, sooner growing tired, and relaxing at the slightest disturbance of nutrition. Indeed, if we inhale the vapour of a substance which, like that of nitrite of amyl, paralyses the blood-vessels, the face immediately becomes of a vivid red, and anyone making this experiment feels his face aflame in a few seconds. This is the simplest method which we possess for artificially producing the external phenomena of shame.

At different ages and in different persons considerable differences are noticeable with regard to the greater or lesser facility with which they blush or grow pale. I made a long series of investigations in order to see at what degree of temperature the paralysis of the blood-vessels of the hands appears when we dip them into hot water, and at what degree, and after what lapse of time, the hands begin to redden when we hold them in ice-water or in snow, the differences being found to be very considerable.

An old lady does not blush under those moral emotions which used to betray her feelings as a girl; and this, not because age has overcome the timidity of youth, or because the hard struggles of life have blunted her sensibility, but because the blood-vessels of the face have, in course of time, become less yielding. On long walks taken in the sun, one always notices that the faces of babies are redder than those of bigger children, and these, in their turn, are more flushed than those of their parents.

Even persons of the same age do not respond in the same way to the internal or external stimuli which tend to dilate or contract the blood-vessels. It is well-known that all girls do not blush equally at a pleasantry directed to them.

One must not ascribe the difference solely to shyness or modesty, since the blood-vessels of different persons respond in various ways. In a very warm room all the young girls have not equally flushed cheeks, and if we pay attention when, on leaving a company, we touch the hands of a great number of people who have been together for several hours in the same room, we may easily notice the very great difference in the temperature of the hands. In such circumstances, to have warm or cold hands only means to have expanded or contracted blood-vessels.

Besides this action of warmth or cold, which is, so to speak, local, there is another central action much more important to us—that which produces the pallor, or flush of emotion. The nerve-centres can, by means of the vaso-motor nerves, greatly alter the circulation in the various parts of the body, as we all know from the continual changes which the colour of the skin undergoes.

It is not necessary to mention the studies made on animals; the observations which can be made on man suffice to show how this nervous mechanism works. I know several persons whose blood-vessels differ in sensitiveness on the right and left side, and who, therefore, feel the effects of emotion more intensely on one side of the body.

At balls, on excursions in the mountains, and walks in the sunshine, the attentive observer will notice great differences in the colour of the two sides of the face. One often becomes aware of this from the perspiration, which is more abundant on one part of the forehead than on the other. My sister, for instance, when dancing, has one cheek very much flushed, the other less so. With her, it is the right side of the body which possesses more sensitive blood-vessels, which are, therefore, more easily tired by exertion, heat, or emotion; consequently this half of the face becomes redder, and receives a greater quantity of blood.

A few days ago we went for a walk together into the mountains. Looking down from a certain point we saw in the valley the funeral of a child. A girl carried the little corpse, covered with flowers, on her head. The bells of the village were ringing the 'Gloria,' the funeral train, with the priest at the head, appeared and vanished from time to time between the green trees; children ran behind, carrying candles and scattering flowers. It was a splendid autumn evening.

We had seen that little cherub with its golden hair just a few days before, healthy and beautiful, enjoying itself at play, and now it was to be hidden for ever under the cypresses of the churchyard. It was our maid who carried the little one on her head; as she had said to us, 'I must take him to be buried, because I am his godmother.'

My sister told me that as she watched she felt a shiver, as though she had goose-skin all down the right side of the body, from head to foot.

Generally, the excitability of the vaso-motor nerves is the same in both halves of the body, and we all experience during strong emotions a feeling of cold, due to the contraction of the vessels, and spreading over the whole body, as though a cold sheet were being wrapped round our limbs and pressed upon our heart; this giving us an impression which one might call a mingling of several indefinite and varying impressions, as of darkness, cold, and of a dull, deep noise. The impression is generally more perceptible in the head and back, more rarely in the legs. Sometimes these contractions of the vessels take place without our knowing the cause; the popular superstition says that death is loitering near. It is one of those contractions arising spontaneously, like the involuntary, sudden starts to which we are often subject in bed before falling asleep.

II

Until recently no one had thought of studying the circulation in hands or feet, since even the most practised eye cannot with certainty distinguish the minimum variations in the colour of the skin, and because the thermometer applied to the surface of the body cannot accurately measure it. It occurred to me that one might easily attain this object by measuring the volume of the hand. I took a long, narrow bottle, and broke out the bottom of it. Into it the hand and a good part of the fore-arm must be introduced, and the bottle closed hermetically with putty. In the neck of the bottle I fastened a stopper, through which a long slender glass tube passed, and filled bottle and glass tube with tepid water.

I thought if a greater quantity of blood flows into the hand, an amount of water corresponding to the increased quantity of blood will be forced out of the bottle, and, on the contrary, if the blood-vessels contract and the hand becomes smaller, the water contained in the slender tube which passes through the stopper will flow into the bottle.

The first experiment, which I made on my brother, convinced me at once that I had discovered the right method, although at that time I was very far from imagining that I should be able to raise my simple apparatus to the dignity of a scientific method, and with it to add a chapter to the treatises of physiology.

I shall not detain the reader with a description of the perfecting of this instrument, to which I gave the name of plethysmograph, or meter of changes of volume.

A few months after making the first experiments on my brother, I returned to Leipzig to see the celebrated physiologist Ludwig, in order to tell him that I had thought out a very simple instrument, by means of which interesting circumstances in the circulation of the blood in man might be noticed. I shall always remember with deep emotion the satisfied look with which he examined the sketches which I, with trembling hand, drew upon the paper in order to make myself intelligible, his sincere pleasure, and the words with which he encouraged me to complete my studies in his laboratory.

I went to work at once and constructed two apparatus, one for each arm, with the intention of studying the circulation in two parts of the body at the same time. The phenomenon which had most surprised me in my first experiments in Italy was the great instability of the blood-vessels of the hand, in consequence of which it changed in volume under the slightest emotions in the most surprising manner, whether the subject were awake or asleep. A few days after having installed myself in the laboratory in Leipzig, I was making an experiment in a room near that of the professor, my colleague, Professor Luigi Pagliani, helping me in everything with the devotion of a friend.

Our first object was to establish the relation between respiration and change of volume in the hands. While Professor Pagliani was standing before the registering apparatus, with his arms in the glass cylinders filled with water, Professor Ludwig walked into the room. Immediately the two pens indicating the volume of the arms, descended, as though a vertical line, ten centimetres in length, were drawn down this page. It was the first time that I had seen such a considerable decrease in the volume of the hand and fore-arm, produced by an apparently slight emotion. Professor Ludwig himself was very much astonished, and, with that affability which made him so beloved by his pupils, took a pen and wrote on the paper at that point where the plethysmograph had marked the disturbance in the circulation caused by his appearance, *Der Löwe kommt* ('Enter the lion').

III

In order to show more clearly the perpetual changes of locality which the blood undergoes, accumulating now in one, now in another part of the body, I constructed a balance of such a size that the beam (made of wood) was sufficiently long and broad to allow of a man's lying at full length upon it, as may be seen in fig. 2. By means of the weights, *R*, which run along the edge of the couch (moving upon the fulcrum, *E*), it is easy, when the centre of gravity of the body is nearly in the middle of the balance, to keep a man in equilibrium. In order to prevent the balance swaying from side to side at every little oscillation, I had to affix a heavy counterpoise of metal, *I*, which can be moved up or down upon the screw, *G H*, fixed vertically in the middle of the plank, *D C*, and firmly held by the lateral bars, *M L*.

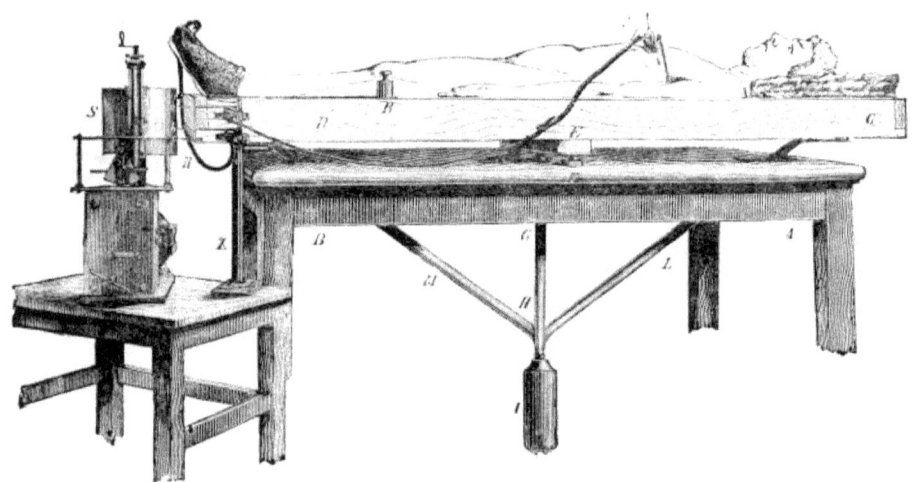

FIG. 2. BALANCE FOR THE STUDY OF THE CIRCULATION OF THE BLOOD IN MAN

The centre of gravity of the balance is placed in this way so low down that it no longer sways at every little oscillation, the counterpoise, which moves inversely to the inclination of the balance, by its weight drawing the plank with it, and bringing it again into a horizontal position. I made the balance so sensitive that it oscillated according to the rhythm of respiration.

If one speaks to a person while he is lying on the balance horizontally, in equilibrium and perfectly quiet, it inclines immediately towards the head. The legs become lighter and the head heavier. This phenomenon is constant, whatever pains the subject may take not to move, however he may endeavour not to alter his breathing, to suspend it temporarily, not to speak, to do nothing which may produce a more copious flow of blood to the brain.

It was always a pleasant sight to my colleagues, visiting me during my researches, when they found some friend or acquaintance sleeping on the balance. In the afternoon hours, which I preferred for my investigations, it often happened that one of them would grow drowsy, and be rocked to sleep by the uniform oscillation of this scientific cradle. Scarcely had some one about to enter touched the handle of the door, than the balance inclined towards the head, remaining immovable in this position for five, six, and even ten minutes, according to the disturbance produced in the sleep. Often, after waking, the blood was no longer distributed in the same manner; the weight R had to be moved towards the feet, from which an amount of blood had retreated in order to circulate more actively in the brain. The subject would then gradually grow drowsy again, and the balance incline towards the feet, the blood flowing, so to speak, from the centres of activity, and collecting in the veins of the feet. The weight R had now to be moved in the opposite direction, until, in sound sleep, that distribution of the blood took place which is peculiar to this state of our organism. In the meantime the respiratory oscillations continued. Then, when all was quiet, one of us would intentionally make a slight noise, by coughing, scraping a foot on the ground, or moving a chair, and at once the balance inclined again towards the head, remaining immovable for four or five minutes, without the subject's noticing anything or awaking. And also, when all was silent in the still hours of night, or during an afternoon sleep, one often noticed, without the appearance of any external cause, oscillations, as it were spontaneous changes of locality of the blood, arising from dreams or psychic conditions acting on the vaso-motor nerves and modifying the circulation, without the participation of consciousness, or at least without a trace of these processes remaining in the memory.

IV

It was proved by my balance that, at the slightest emotion, the blood rushes to the head. But this did not satisfy me. I wished to analyse this phenomenon more minutely, and constructed other new instruments in order to study it in all its particulars, and to follow the blood while it streams from hands, feet, and arms to the brain. I have traced the pulse for hours together, not of one part only, but nearly always of several parts of the body at the same time—of the brain, the hands, the feet, noting the slightest changes which the activity of thought, external impressions, noises, or dreams produced on the blood-vessels, waking or sleeping.

It was already known that the pulsations of the heart augment under the influence of food and drink, but no one had observed, by means of other instruments, certain modifications which the form of the pulse undergoes, and which are so characteristic that I need now only see the curve of a single pulsation of hand or foot in order to know whether the person had eaten or was fasting. Again, between two pulsations presented to me, I can distinguish that of the thinking and that of the absent-minded man, that of the sleeper and that of one awake, that of one who is warm and that of one who is cold, that of the tired man and that of him who has rested, that of one who is afraid and that of one who is tranquil.

One of my literary friends came one day to visit me in the laboratory, in order to convince himself with his own eyes of these results, which seemed to him scarcely credible. I proposed to make an experiment upon himself, to see whether any change would be observable in his pulse when he passed from reading an Italian book to a Greek one. At first he laughed at the idea, but when we put it to the proof, we found that with him also the pulse of the wrist changed considerably when he passed from an easy work to the more difficult one of translating, unprepared, a passage from Homer.

The vital processes are the more active the greater the rapidity with which the blood circulates in our body; but in order to accelerate the movement of the blood, the blood-vessels must contract. What we notice in the course of rivers, namely, that the current becomes quicker at that point where the bed is narrower, takes place also in our circulatory system. When we are threatened by a danger, during fear, emotion, when the organism must develop its strength, an automatic contraction of the blood-vessels takes place, which renders the movement of the blood more rapid in the nerve-centres.

It is on this account that the vessels at the surface of the body contract, and we grow pale from fright or during violent emotion. I have measured exactly the amount of blood which retreats from hands and feet during the slightest emotions, also the number of seconds between the moment when the emotion arises and that when the pallor is greatest, but this is not the place for statistics.

A gentleman once told me that from fright a ring had one day fallen from his finger which at other times he could only remove with difficulty. He had also noticed that his fingers actually grew smaller whenever he experienced strong emotion, thus rendering it easier to take off the ring.

The proverb, 'Cold hand, warm heart,' is the popular expression of the fact that the hands grow cold when the blood, in consequence of an emotion, retreats from the limbs to the heart.

CHAPTER VI

THE BEATING OF THE HEART

I

In all ages and by all peoples the heart has been looked upon as the centre of the passions, of feeling and of strength. Our word courage comes from 'cœur'—heart. Nearly two thousand years ago it was proved by physiologists that the heart was not the centre of sensibility, and yet poets and common opinion continue to say that the heart is the most sensitive part of the body.

In August 1879 Biffi showed in the Instituto Lombardo the heart of a youth, in the left wall of which, in the autopsy, he had found a needle sticking. The youth, who was of good family, was a poor unfortunate who had killed his father in a fit of insanity, had then tried repeatedly to commit suicide, and at length died mad in the hospital. While he was still living with his family, about two years before his death, he had said that he had stuck a needle into his heart, in order to put an end to his life, but no one believed him. During the whole time which he spent in the hospital the movements of the heart were regular and quiet, the pulse normal, respiration easy, sleep good; he could lie in all positions, and he never complained of any oppression in the region of the heart. When he was dead a needle with a rusted eye was found buried in the flesh and covered with a sheath which had grown around it; the sharp, polished point had penetrated into the cavity of the heart. The irritation caused by the perpetual pricking had produced fleshy excrescences at that point where the heart was continually grazed.

This instance shows how insensible the heart is, and yet, in the language of the poets and in the imagination of the people, it will always remain the centre of the passions and of feeling, because during fear, and in the decisive moments of life, we feel it hammering against the walls of the chest like a machine hidden within, the force of its contractions booming and echoing in our ears and head, exciting that strange feeling of oppression which we imagine that this rebellious organ, unchained by a storm of passion, alone produces.

The heart is nothing but a force-pump situated in the centre of the blood-vessels, which, by the play of its valves and the contractions of its muscles, keeps up the circulation in arteries and veins, driving the blood into all parts of the body, an arrangement without which life would be impossible.

II

In studying a machine one first seeks the most important part, without which it could not move nor work. In the mechanism of our body, the first part to develop and move is the heart, and it likewise is the last to stand still. The development of this organ may be better studied in the hen's egg than in any other animal, as it can be seen on the second day of incubation. At its first appearance it is in man, as in animals, a fine, curved tube in the shape of an **S**. If we break an egg taken from under a brood-hen towards the end of the second or the beginning of the third day, the first rudiment of the heart may already be seen pulsating. Towards the end of the fourth week after conception, the human heart has already nearly the form which it preserves during the whole of life. It is wonderful with what resistance the heart struggles on its first appearance against every cause which threatens its life. Professor Pflüger relates that a human embryo of about three weeks' gestation was left a whole night between two watch-glasses in a cold room. In the morning it was found that the little heart still contracted at intervals of twenty to thirty seconds, and these movements were noticeable for almost another hour, becoming gradually slower and weaker until the complete death of the embryo.

In animals incompletely developed there is no emotion capable of modifying the rhythm of the heart. In a series of experiments which I made on the heart in a hen's egg during the first days of its development, I found that the application of the strongest inductive currents, such as were unbearable on the hands, produced not the least effect. It was a strange sight, this surprising tenacity and unexpected resistance in a little heart which was scarcely visible, and which pulsated tranquilly under electrical discharges which would have killed instantaneously the heart of a horse or an ox.

This shows us how well the organs are adapted to their functions. It is the task of the heart in the chicken to work blindly and incessantly in order to bring into circulation the little particles which gradually build up the body of the animal, using for this purpose the materials accumulated in the egg after it has received the spark of life through fecundation. In the embryo there is no need to receive the impressions of the outside world, and the organs for this purpose are still lacking, the nerves have not yet appeared, the heart is free in the midst of the chaos of matter in the course of organisation.

III

The fully-developed heart has a much more complicated innervation than the other muscles. The arm or leg cut off from the body ceases at once to move, but the heart removed from an animal continues to beat for a long time. Those who frequent the anatomical lecture-rooms notice sometimes with surprise slight movements at the base of the heart, although the rest of the corpse has been cold and motionless for a whole day. The heart owes this tenacity of life to the structure of its thin walls, to its being immersed in blood, and, more than all, to there being in its flesh little nerve-centres called ganglia. It is on this account, however, by no means independent of the brain and spinal cord, which can modify the rhythm and force of its pulsations according to the needs of the internal economy. Our organism is one of the most wonderful examples of that happy autonomy where liberty and the functions of each organ are always subordinated to the interest and advantage of all others, while the joint administration has as its object the maintenance of life and the welfare of all.

The centre of the cardiac nerves is in the medulla oblongata, in the most important part of the nervous system, near that point the wounding of which even with a pin-point causes instant death, because there all the paths of the nervous system converge.

Of the two nerves which carry commands to the heart, one serves principally to slacken the pulsations, and has, since it acts as a brake, received the name of inhibitory nerve; while the other, serving to increase the frequency of the beats, to spur them on, so to speak, is called the accelerator nerve.

The functions of the cardiac nerves, which may seem in this way to be extremely simple, are in reality very complicated. Galvani was the first who showed that an irritation of the spinal cord brought about an arrest, or, as he called it, an *enchantment* (*incantesimo*) of the heart.

IV

Boccaccio describes in a masterly manner the effects and changes which love produces on the pulse:

'Thus it happened that he sickened most seriously through excess of passion. Then were several physicians called to restore him, but, despite their careful watching, they could not guess his disease, and despaired of his recovery. And so it came to pass that one day, while a physician, still young indeed, but of profound science, sat near the patient, holding his arm there where the pulse beats, Giannetta came for some reason into the room where the youth was lying, who, when he saw the maiden, did not indeed betray his emotion either by word or gesture, but felt the ardour of passion increase in his heart, wherefore his pulse began to beat more violently than before. This the physician incontinently noticed and wondered, but remained still to see how long these pulsations would continue. When Giannetta left the room, the pulse became calmer. The physician, now deeming he had discovered the reason of the malady, caused the maiden to be called on the pretext of having a question to put to her, he still holding the patient by the wrist. Scarcely had she come into the room than the youth's pulse beat more rapidly, slackening once more at her departure. Whereupon the physician, believing himself in possession of the truth, arose, and taking the parents of the young man aside, said to them: "The health of your son needs not the physician's art; it lies in Giannetta's hands."'

So Boccaccio describes the diagnosis of the illness of the Count of Antwerp; and long before Boccaccio, Plutarch had already stated that the physician Erasistratus discovered the love of Antiochus to Stratonice from the tumultuous irregularity of his pulse.

We here touch upon one of the greatest problems which criminal science will propound in the future, when it asks the physiologist: 'Tell us of what does this man think, who remains impassive before the traces of his crime? Tell us if within him there is nothing pulsating—nothing, either human or animal?'

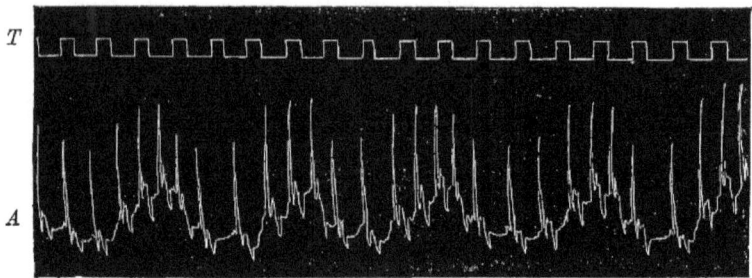

FIG. 3.—CURVE SHOWING CARDIAC PULSATIONS OF A QUIET DOG

I have in my laboratory a dog which was of service to me in a few studies on fatigue. He is such a good animal that for two years I have kept him, together with two other dogs of which I have grown fond, and which, like old friends, shall always stay with me, unless some dog-lover comes to beg them from me, as so often happens with good, faithful dogs, that only in the physiological laboratories can escape from the certain and cruel death to which the Corporation condemns them. As he is a quiet dog, it occurred to me one day to try the effect of a violent noise upon him. I made use of a little instrument called a *cardiograph*, because it transmits the heart-beats to a lever which traces them on a cylinder covered with smoked paper. I applied this instrument, which is about the size of a half-crown, on the place where the heart beats between the ribs, fixing it by means of an elastic band fastened round the thorax. At first it wrote the curve of the cardiac pulsations represented in fig. 3, which is reproduced by means of photozincography. I regret having to present the reader with more curves, but when one is able to see what the heart itself writes, it would be unpardonable to try to translate its characteristic language into words. Besides, it is not difficult to understand these curves. The line T signifies the time; it is written by an electric clock which raises a pen every second and marks a tooth. It is, so to speak, a controlling line, indispensable in graphic studies by which one wishes to learn with the greatest exactness the changes which the frequency of the pulse undergoes. In the line T eighteen seconds are marked, and the heart-beats registered in the same time in line A amount to twenty-nine. If I had applied the cardiograph to the thorax of a man I should have obtained a similar curve with fewer pulsations. At each beat of the heart the pen rises and falls rapidly, and then writes below a trembling line during which the heart does not beat. As the thorax rises and expands during inspiration, the pen resting on the ribs must likewise rise, therefore the three or four pulsations taking place during the expansion of the thorax are marked successively higher, sinking again with the commencement of expiration, thus forming waves, as it were. From this curve, traced while the animal was tranquil, we see that its heart, as indeed is also the case in man, beats more frequently during inspiration than during expiration, the heart-beats being nearer to each other in the ascending portion of the curve, and further apart in the lower portion which corresponds to the end of each expiration.

While the animal was perfectly quiet I motioned to my servant to fire a gun, but he failed. It was an old hunting-gun, badly loaded perhaps, and only the cartridge had caught fire. The dog, however, at once tried to rise, and became strangely excited, much to our surprise. I had my hands on the instrument which lay on the ribs where the heart beats, and felt that its palpitations had become stronger and more rapid. About a minute later we succeeded in taking the curve *B* in fig. 4, from which may be seen how much more frequent the pulsations were. The animal had become so restless that we had to give up the experiment and set him at liberty. When he was on the ground he went round the laboratory sniffing everywhere. Presently we took the curve *C*, fig. 4, from which we can see that the emotion was not yet over, since the beating of the heart is still quicker than in the normal curve marked in fig. 3.

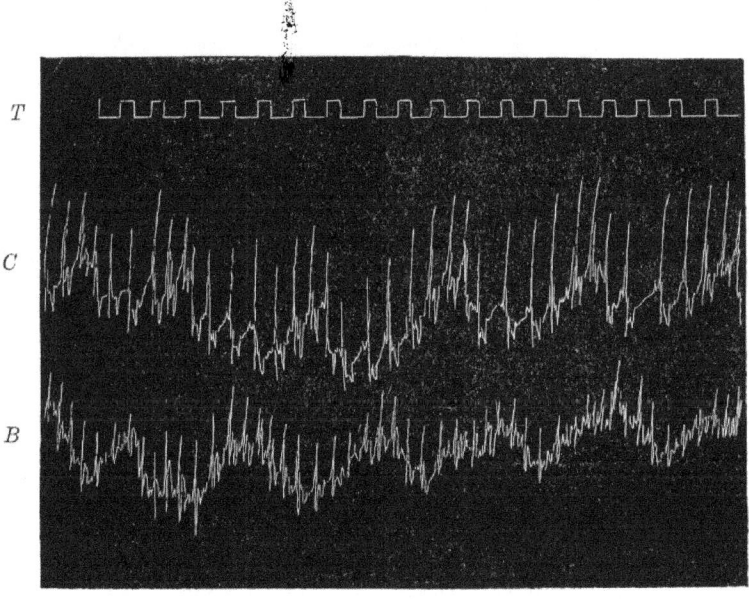

FIG. 4.—CARDIAC PULSATION DURING EMOTION

There were several of us together when this experiment was made—the students of the laboratory, my assistants, and Professor Corona, and we were all astonished at what took place. Some of the bystanders said at once that it must be a hound. We had always taken him for a watch-dog, as he was very big, and did not look in the least like a hound. We determined to try a decisive experiment the next day.

We waited till the animal was perfectly quiet, and then held a gun so that he could see it at a distance of a few steps from him, without threatening him in any way. The dog at once recognised the weapon, and again grew excited, showing a considerable change in the cardiac curve.

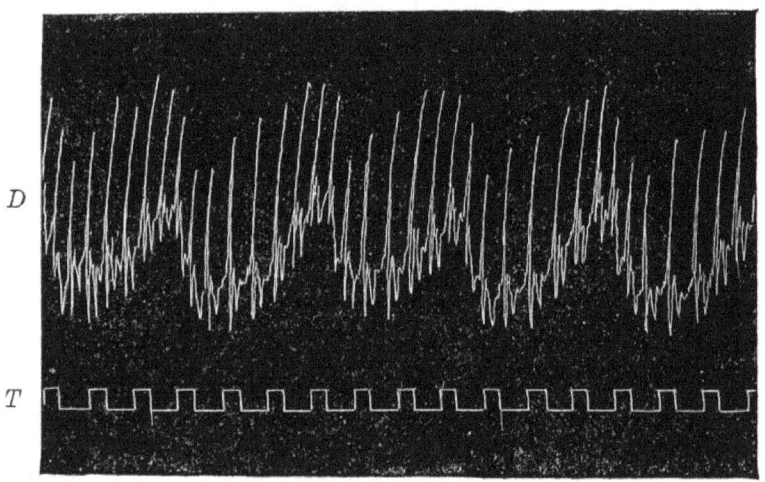

FIG. 5.—NORMAL CARDIAC PULSATION

But the most evident proof that it was a hound was given by the very violent emotion and the unexpected excitement which took possession of him as soon as he heard the noise caused by the loading of the gun and the click of the trigger. Even when he saw nothing, and this noise was made at some distance from him, the beating of the heart changed instantly (as may be seen in the following curve), and the animal tried to rise and sniffed the air.

The curve D, fig. 5, shows the pulsations written with the cardiograph applied to the thorax of the animal when quiet.

At a given time I signed to a person, whom the dog could not see, to load the gun. Scarcely had the animal heard the clicking than he moved; a few seconds passed, during which it was impossible to take the curve, the dog being so restless. About a minute later I succeeded in obtaining the curve E, fig. 6, in which one can see that the form of respiration, as well as the frequency and force of the cardiac pulsations, is altered.

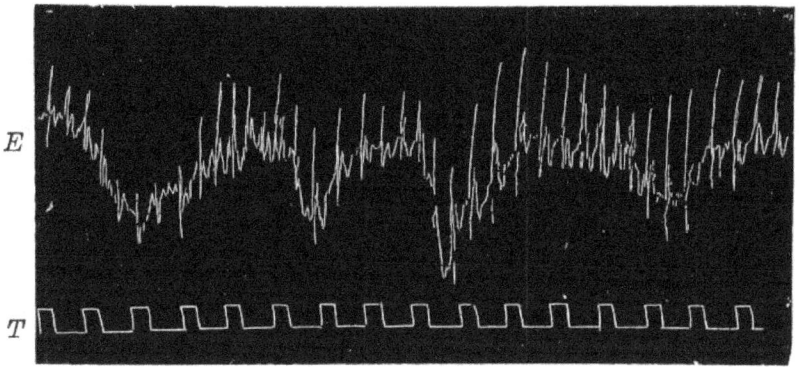

FIG. 6.—ALTERATION OF THE CARDIAC PULSATION THROUGH EMOTION

After we had assured ourselves that these alterations of the pulse were much less marked after other noises which did not resemble the loading of a gun, we wished to convince ourselves whether the agitation was caused by a fear of weapons. The next day the dog was again brought into the laboratory, and while he lay on the table, and the action of the heart was being marked, someone walked past him with a gun on his shoulder. The dog recognised it again, became restless, tried to rise, his heart beat violently, he began to wag his tail, and followed the hunter with satisfied glances.

V

When strong emotions such as fear are concerned, one must have recourse to other methods of writing the pulse, as the animal is very uneasy and tries to escape. As this is a question as yet little considered in physiology, I shall communicate a few experiments which I made bearing upon it. Fig. 7 represents the pulse of the carotid artery of a dog. During line *F* the animal was quiet; the pulse is somewhat irregular, which, in the dog, is a physiological fact. In line *G* five normal pulsations may be seen, while at *A* a shot was fired two steps from the dog. The report caused such a vibration of the air that the pen trembled, as may be seen from the irregular outline of the first two pulsations. The effect of fear on the heart is immediate. The frequency of the beats becomes at once three times greater than before.

We waited till the dog was quiet again. Fifteen minutes afterwards the curve *H*, which represents the normal pulse-line, was written, then came six pulsations of the line *I*, while at *B* a second shot was fired, and immediately the pulse was accelerated.

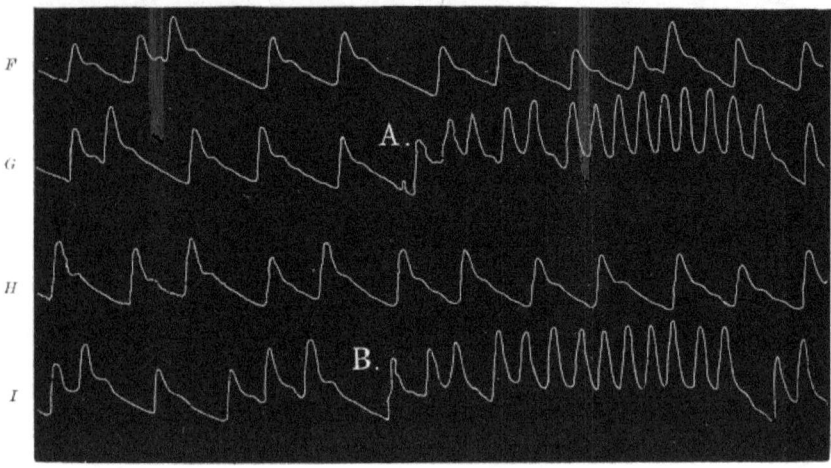

FIG. 7.—ACCELERATION OF THE CARDIAC PULSATIONS THROUGH FEAR

(IN A AND B)

But why does the heart beat more rapidly and frequently in fear? In order to explain the cause of this phenomenon I must remind the reader of the observations which I made during my studies of the pulse, and of the circulation of the blood in the human brain during sleep. In a sleeping person, at the slightest noise or touch, the pulse becomes more frequent without the sleep being interrupted. This change is indispensable in order to accelerate the circulation and to utilise to the utmost the strength of the organism in preparing it for defence. Our machine is so made that it changes automatically as required, without the interference of the will being necessary. The palpitation of the heart from fear is the exaggeration of a fact which we always notice, whenever the organism must develop its maximum of energy and increase the circulation in the nerve-centres; the heart does not work for itself, but for the brain and muscles, which are the instruments of combat, attack, defence, and flight.

The greater or lesser frequency and force of the pulse in emotion depends upon the greater or lesser excitability of the nerve-centres. Women and children, who are more sensitive, experience this palpitation in greater intensity. When we say that women have more tender hearts, we refer to the fact that their hearts respond to stimuli to which the hearts of men remain impassive. We say of anyone who blushes and grows pale easily, and is soon moved to tears or laughter, that he has a good heart and a sincere character. But even cold, sceptical, egotistic, impassive men, when they are suffering from some illness, or when the excitability of their nervous system is intensified by some cause or other, may be deeply moved, and betray their feelings like children.

64

One must be a physician in order to see how the most courageous men become faint-hearted at a trifling loss of blood, and timid people, in consequence of a more abundant flow of blood to the brain, perform miracles of bravery. Weakness quickens the heart-beat even when we are not moved by anything. We all know that we avoid giving certain news to the convalescent which at other times would have produced little effect upon them.

One of my colleagues had been ill eight days from a quinsy. When he recovered and came to the laboratory, I hastened to visit him, and found him sitting in an arm-chair, pale and exhausted. I asked him how he was, to which he answered 'Very well,' but that while scolding his servant on account of some trifling matter, such a feeling of oppression had seized him that he had to desist, as he was scarcely able to draw breath. I felt his pulse, and found that it was above a hundred. He laughed, and said, 'I never dreamt that my strong body was such a paltry piece of machinery as to run down during the few days I have not eaten as usual.'

VI

It is necessary for the heart, as for all muscles, to be fed. For it, indeed, this need is more imperative, as it may not stand still in order to rest when it is tired. The continuous work to which it is condemned explains to us how every alteration in the composition and amount of blood is immediately manifested by changing its nutrition and consequently its strength. Knowing that the heart is in constant contact with the blood, that is, with the nutriment distributed by it to all parts of the body, one might think that it could in this way take the best part for itself, as it helps itself at first hand; at the least, that it would take a more abundant portion than the other organs, or that nature allowed it to satisfy its appetite unreservedly. But this is not the case. In our body the rations of all organs are calculated and distributed according to the need of each. There is also a very strict economy of nutrition observed, because when any part of the body works more than usual, its increased needs are supplied by diminishing the rations of the other organs. The vaso-motor nerves are charged with this distribution of victuals, if I may so express myself. The heart, like all other muscles, takes as much blood as it needs for its maintenance out of its cavity by means of the coronary arteries branching off from the aorta. There is a control exercised over the heart also, and the vaso-motor nerves could, if it were absolutely necessary, diminish its rations and leave it barely sufficient strength to distribute the food to all the other parts of the body.

Physiologists have endeavoured in vain during the last centuries to find in the greater or lesser nutrition of the cardiac muscle the cause of its more or less accelerated movements. One of the most daring theories was propounded by Giovanni Lancisi, the celebrated Roman court-physician, one of the most illustrious physiologists Italy has ever possessed.

In his book 'De motu cordis,' printed in the year 1728 by the Roman University Press, he develops a theory so manifestly materialistic of the origin of the pulsation of the heart during emotion and mental suffering, that it seems almost impossible the book should have been dedicated to the memory of Clement XI. and printed with the pontifical types, by permission of the Sacred College. The Roman curia did not foresee that those first steps would lead physiology so far away from their dogmas, and did not suspect that such simple notions about the functions of the human machine were pregnant with the innovative germs of modern philosophy, since it allowed its great physician to speak freely, and since it furnished him with the means for his physiological investigations, heaped honours upon him, and handed down splendid editions of his immortal books to posterity.

Mental functions are placed by Lancisi in close dependence on the nerves, the ganglia, and the coronary vessels of the heart. The material organs it is which influence mental movements. The heat of passion, the storm of emotions, have in the heart mechanisms by which they may be moderated and regulated. It is as though the nerves and ganglia of the heart, by driving the blood with more or less violence into the brain, could excite the instincts; as though the character and disposition of the mind depended on the material structure and the physical modifications of the body.

CHAPTER VII

RESPIRATION AND OPPRESSION

I

Oppression on the chest has in it something so irresistible that the will cannot subdue it. A slight emotion, a little exertion, a loss of blood, or a fever is sufficient, nay, it is only necessary to enter a room where the air is warm or bad, to stoop or to go up steps, in order at once to accelerate the breath. So long as we are quiet, we may believe ourselves able to modify our respiratory movements at will; but, when the calm ceases, the working of our machine becomes apparent, and we are no longer able to arrest it. Our liberty is in no respect complete with regard to the functions of the organism. We are like children whom Nature allows to play so long as there is no danger to life.

In order to understand the meaning of the continual variations which respiration undergoes, we must remember that our body is a very complicated furnace, in which, to keep the flame of life aglow, something must constantly be burnt. The respiratory movements, the expansion and contraction of the lungs, represent the untiring work of a bellows which keeps up the fire in the smithy of our organism. We may breathe in two ways: either we expand the upper part of the thorax by raising the ribs, or we expand it lower down by depressing the diaphragm. The first movement is more common with women, in whom the rise and fall of the bosom during emotion is so characteristic; the other is more usual with men. When we sleep it is especially the diaphragm which reposes; with some persons the abdomen is almost motionless during sleep, but a slight noise or push, a voice, or any external action suffices to make it resume its functions, and the diaphragmatic breathing becomes more active. This takes place suddenly, without our waking or being aware of it, and without any recollection of it remaining in consciousness.

After this slight uneasiness, during which sleep becomes lighter for a few minutes, is past, the respiration resumes the rhythm and characteristic form of deep sleep. These changes, which take place without any participation of the will, form one of the most wonderful arrangements observable in this perfect machine of ours. When we lose consciousness, Nature could not expose our body to the influences of the external world, leaving it defenceless, a prey to dangerous enemies. It is necessary that a detachment of the nerve-centres should, even during sleep, keep watch on the outside world, and in good time prepare the material conditions of consciousness and the attitude of resistance. All unconscious phenomena which I have seen appear in the transition from sleeping to waking are destined to increase the circulation of the blood in the brain and reanimate the functions and energy of the body. These centres are sentinels on the defensive, watching continually and sounding the alarm when danger is nigh.

Man falls asleep after the labours of the day. The muscles relax, head and arms fall powerless, the lids droop and cover the eyes, the legs no longer hold us erect. The feverish waking activity ceases, the fire slackens gradually within us, combustion is so much less active, that the respiratory movements, which, during calm, waking moments introduce about seven litres of air into the lungs every minute, have now reduced the ventilation to one litre per minute. The heart, too, rests by lessening the frequency of its contractions and diminishing the energy and extent of the systole; the vessels enlarge, the pressure of blood falls, and the body becomes noticeably colder. But, in spite of this loss of consciousness and complete relaxation of the body, there is still a close net of nerves and masses of nerve-cells which retain their energy and watch over us. A voice, a distant noise, a ray of light, a slight touch, any impression is enough to rouse the bellows to renewed activity, to double the number of heart-beats, to cause the vessels of the whole surface of the skin to contract, thus driving the blood to the centres of life and restoring the material conditions of consciousness.

In the struggle for existence that organism will most easily escape the injuries of the external world in which this unconscious vigilance is most perfect, and which is able with the greatest promptitude to pass from the condition of profound repose to that of greatest activity before the danger comes too near and injury is inevitable.

II

These studies of mine of the respiration in sleeping and waking man make us understand more readily the signification of oppression during emotion. The difference is only one of intensity and degree, not of the nature and quality of the phenomenon. There is the same relation between waking and sleeping as between calm and agitation of mind. Let us consider the proof of this.

If we wish to study the respiratory movements with great accuracy, it is no longer sufficient to observe how the thorax expands and contracts; we must apply to chest and abdomen extremely delicate instruments which mark automatically the slightest motion of the thorax. These instruments, called *pneumographs*, are made in such a manner as to cause no annoyance to the person on whom they are applied. I shall communicate a few observations which I made on my dog. He is such a good animal, that when I apply the pneumograph to the thorax and put him on the table in order to write the respiratory movements, he lies for hours quietly slumbering. But a mere nothing, the slightest noise, is sufficient to cause an alteration in the rhythm of breathing. This is an experiment which I have often repeated before my colleagues, in order to show the extreme sensibility of the respiratory mechanism to psychic conditions.

While all was quiet and the pneumograph was writing the respiratory curve, it was enough if I spoke to someone, if I gave an order, touched the apparatus or the table, or even if I looked at the dog and spoke kindly to him—his breathing immediately became more rapid.

If the impression were slight, the effect lasted a few seconds; sometimes I found that a single respiration had become quicker, but generally the effect lasted longer. If a person whom the dog did not know placed himself before him, the former respiratory rhythm did not return; if I scolded him, the effect lasted many minutes till the emotion had subsided.

Since I was in the laboratory at Leipzig I have made researches into the changes which cerebral activity exercises on the respiratory movements of men. This is a very complicated problem, as individual differences are great. In the curves which I obtained from some of my colleagues, who kindly placed themselves at my disposition for my observations on respiration, I found that the differences during intense mental work are very considerable. The reason for this must be sought in the variable excitability of the nerve-centres, and especially in the fact that the respiratory mechanism acts in a contrary manner during strong and during weak emotions. I made a few experiments on myself in order to see how the breathing changed, when someone suddenly made a great noise, as, for instance, by firing a gun behind my back while I was reading or absent-minded. I repeated these experiments on dogs, and always found that a deeper, often very deep, inspiration is caused, then there seems to be an arrest of respiration which may last for several seconds, the respiratory movements becoming immediately afterwards more frequent than before. Sometimes in a dog I observed that a shot caused, first, a deep inspiration, then a light expiration and inspiration, while the chest was much expanded; then another deep inspiration like the first, after which the chest emptied itself of the air accumulated in the lungs, and a succession of quicker breaths with more rapid inspirations than usual was drawn. Those who wish to find at once a plausible reason for all phenomena will perhaps say that these deep breaths serve to oxidise and vivify the blood streaming through the lungs, so that in this way the organism may prepare itself for defence.

III

Let us now see of what parts the respiratory machine consists, and how it puts its force into operation. In man the different parts of this mechanism never act sufficiently in independence of each other to allow of our surprising them separately at work. Only after decapitation has the head been seen to make inspiratory movements although separated from the trunk. Physicians who have had to be present at the execution of the condemned tell of the terrible effect produced when the head of the man rolls, gasping, to the ground, becoming instantaneously of a corpse-like pallor, and disfigured by strange, spasmodic contractions, the eyes rolling irregularly, horribly, for several seconds. The trunk is already motionless, the blood, which at first poured forth in great streams from the arteries of the neck, only spurts feebly and at intervals, still obeying the weakening pulsations of the heart. The eyes at last turn upwards, but life is not yet quite extinct, the mouth still opens from time to time as though with a great effort. The inspirations which at first distended the nostrils and opened wide the mouth soon become less distinct and less frequent, until at last they die away altogether.

If, after cutting off the head of a very young animal, we stop the hæmorrhage by means of a bandage and then introduce a bellows into the trachea, so that respiration may be artificially stimulated, we see that the headless animal begins to breathe after the cessation of the perturbing influence of the first shock. With kittens it is sufficient to administer a small dose of strychnine (0·0005 gr.) in order to produce respiratory movements in the trunk after decapitation, which, however, become gradually weaker as they no longer suffice to maintain the excitability of the nerve-centres through the oxidation of the blood.

This simple experiment proves that respiration is accomplished by nerves branching off from the brain and spinal cord. The consciousness of our ego is not necessary; even a decapitated animal responds by modifications of respiration when we pinch or squeeze his paws, because the sensory nerves of the skin transmit the impressions of the external world to the spinal cord. The deep, noisy, and interrupted inspirations of anyone taking a plunge-bath are also involuntary, and when we are overcome by fear it is the same mechanism which produces a deep inspiration.

At every step which physiology makes, we discover fresh complications, other wheels, if I may use the expression, within the wheels of our organism. Until quite recently it was thought that the brain controlled the respiratory centre, accelerating or arresting its movements; but it has now been shown by Christiani that by means of a vivid light which must strike the eyes of the animal, deep and frequent inspirations may be produced even after the brain has been removed. Impressions of sound, which would have frightened the animal, produce the same effect, the oppression being even greater than in normal conditions. This experiment shows us that, independently of cerebral action and psychic operations, the rhythm of breathing alters at every change which takes place in the external world, at every peripheral irritation of the sensory nerves. Thus are explained the oppression and palpitation of the heart which befall us at the banging of a door, at a clap of thunder, and which we cannot suppress, which are produced by a sudden noise on a thousand occasions before we learn the cause, and do not disappear even when we have done so, and recognised the unimportant origin of our perturbation.

In these studies, also, the materiality of psychic processes becomes evident, as well as the slowness of operation in those phenomena which are believed to be the most rapid in life.

Just as an electric spark or a flash of lightning which lasts the one-thousandth part of a second leaves an impression in us a hundred times longer; just as our eye is unable to follow the different positions of a burning brand swung round in the dark, but sees, as it were, a ribbon of fire; just as we burn our hand when we touch a glowing object before we have time to feel the pain; just as, when in movement, we often stumble against obstacles which confront us without our having time to stop; so the impressions which reach the nerve-centres keep us agitated for some time without our having the force to stand still midway on the declivity down which the sudden impetus of the emotion is speeding us. We have all experienced this inability of the organism, we know that we do not succeed in subduing even the slightest mental perturbations. Suppose a person is walking quietly along, when suddenly he sees before him the figure of a man whom he was trying to avoid. At once his blood begins to boil. Scarcely, however, has he seen the man before he becomes aware that he has made a mistake, and he is glad; but his heart has already begun to beat more vigorously, the perturbation and oppression do not at once subside, but continue to annoy for some time. They are like the continued vibrations of a cord that has been shaken, like a flame shooting up as the spark disturbs the equilibrium of the molecules in the nerve-centres, like the echo of a sound reverberating in the nervous fibres and slowly dying away.

IV

What is the last expression of pain, the last manifestation of sensibility? This is a question we must study in order to learn the relative importance of the phenomena making up the picture of fear, and to see which of these offer the most lengthened resistance in the struggle with death.

By means of chloral or alcohol I have produced such a profound sleep in dogs or rabbits that they could not rouse themselves again. One cannot imagine a quieter decease, a gentler and more gradual sinking of the organism into the arms of death.

As soon as a strong dose of chloral or alcohol has been administered, the animal becomes somewhat excited, the hind legs begin to give way; when we call him he cannot turn without falling; he rises, makes another attempt, totters, turns round, falls again, rises with difficulty, and finally lies down stretched out and tranquil. From time to time he tries to raise his head and then falls into a leaden sleep. The respiration is slower, the temperature gradually falls, at length the wagging of the tail ceases. The lids droop over the sleepy eyes, the face is tranquil, the ears motionless, whatever pain the efforts made to awaken him may cause. One might think he was dead.

The only method which physiologists had of finding out whether an animal in this condition was still capable of feeling was by investigating whether the heart and blood-vessels still responded to painful stimuli.

My friend, Professor Foà, showed in a work carried out together with Professor M. Schiff,[14] that even when heart and blood-vessels no longer respond, when the circulation is no longer modified, whatever may be the perturbation of the nerve-

---

[14] Foà e M. Schiff. *La pupilla come estesiometro.* In the *Imparziale,* 1874, p. 617.

centres, a last trace of sensibility may still be observed in the eye, the pupil dilating whenever the animal is irritated.

But I have seen dogs, poisoned with chloral, of which the temperature had sunk to 30°, so extremely slow had the chemical processes of respiration become; no electric current, no mechanical action was capable of producing even the slightest movement of the limbs or face; the pulse, pressure of blood, the pupil, in a word everything had become impassive, no effect being obtained on the pulse even when the cardiac nerves were laid bare, severed, irritated by electric currents—and yet the animal was still sensible. By carefully studying the respiration I saw that it was modified whenever a leg or any other part of the body was pinched.

The alteration of the breathing is therefore the last function of the organism in which sensibility and emotion reveal themselves.

V

We know that, whatever nerve of the skin is irritated, a succession of deeper and more frequent inspirations follows, and we have seen that this phenomenon is useful to the organism. But if the excitement of a nerve becomes so strong as to cause violent pain, or if a very vivid impression is received as in fright, the mechanism stops short midway in a deep inspiration, and this is injurious.

Some few times I have been in danger of my life, and always remember to have felt a terrible oppression, as though my breath had been cut short. A few months ago I was overtaken by a storm on the mountains, when the lightning struck the ground about fifty steps from me, and I remember having noticed that respiration was arrested for several seconds.

We, who carry this fragile machine of our body about with us continually, ought to remember that every shock which exceeds the usual measure may prove fatal. A slight touch of the pendulum accelerates the rotation of the wheels, a stronger one stops their movement; a slight impetus helps us onward, a rude push throws us to the ground. It is thus that the phenomena of fear, which may be useful to us in lesser degrees, become morbid and fatal to the organism as soon as they exceed a certain limit; for this reason fear must be looked upon as a disease.

Most noticeable is this irregularity of respiration in children. We all remember to have seen children fall, and to have remarked with astonishment that, after a shrill scream, they remained still for some time, finally bursting into broken sobs. This is a suspension of respiration. When the sudden pain of a violent blow is felt, the child draws a deep breath with contracted glottis, and emits a sharp cry, then at the height of the inspiration a spasmodic arrest occurs.

There are some very nervous children in whom this spasmodic arrest takes place even in slight emotions. I knew a child of this kind, who, one day, because its father had not taken it with him, began to cry brokenly, and suffered an arrest of breath which lasted a minute or longer. The child's mouth was wide open, he became livid, lips and countenance were purplish, the eyes were half shut and full of tears. The struggle for breath was so great that the child lost its balance and fell, expelled fæces and urine, and then recovered as though nothing had happened. I was told that this took place whenever the child was thwarted.

CHAPTER VIII

TREMBLING

I

The old physiologists believed that the mind of brutes only obeyed two stimuli—pain and pleasure, and that all processes of their organism had as aim to avoid the bad and procure the good. Albrecht von Haller combated this opinion in the last century. 'This theory', he says, 'does not in any way accord with the phenomena. If you consider the movements of an animal during fear, in imminent danger, as having preservation of life for their object, is there anything more absurd than the trembling of the knees and the sudden weakness which befalls it? I am persuaded that all phenomena of fear common to animals are not aimed at the preservation of the timid but rather at their destruction. In order to preserve a just balance it is necessary that the more prolific animals should be destroyed by the less prolific, therefore necessary that those animals destined to be the prey of others should not be able to defend themselves easily'.[15]

I think Charles Darwin must not have been acquainted with this explanation of trembling, as I am convinced he would otherwise have tried to combat it, or would at least have mentioned it in his writings. He was much too conscientious to ignore an objection made to his theories.

Here we have the example of another phenomenon which seems to contradict certain hypotheses of Spencer and Darwin. If it is true that, in the struggle for existence, animals have always perfected those capabilities which are most useful to them in defending themselves, and have gradually left behind, with the generations that have succumbed, all dispositions of the organism which were pernicious to the preservation of the species, why have they not succeeded in freeing themselves from trembling? Why, on the contrary, in critical, decisive moments, when danger confronts them, when their existence is threatened, when nothing is more imperative than flight, attack or defence, do we see animals paralysed with trembling, incapable of struggling, and perishing without their strength having in the least profited them? As Haller's hypothesis is not sufficient to justify such a serious imperfection in organisms, we must seek the reasons and causes of this phenomenon elsewhere.

II

Charles Darwin, in his celebrated book on the 'Expression of the Emotions,' says: 'Trembling, which is common to man and to many, or most, of the lower animals, is

---

[15] Haller: *Elementa physiologiæ corporis humani,* tom. v., lib. xvii. § vii.

of no service, often of much disservice, and cannot have been at first acquired through the will, and then rendered habitual in association with any emotion.'[16] He then remarks that trembling is a very obscure phenomenon, and drops the subject.

Paolo Mantegazza accuses Darwin of great negligence with regard to this important problem, and says in his estimable work on 'Physiognomy and Mimicry,' 'Darwin confesses that he does not consider trembling during fear useful; but, according to my experimental studies of pain, I find it most serviceable, as it tends to generate warmth, to heat the blood which is inclined to grow too cold under the influence of fear.'[17]

Since I must take part in this controversy, there is no other way but to examine attentively the various conditions of the organism in which trembling occurs, and then discuss the matter without prejudice. I acknowledge that I approach this task with some trepidation, because Mantegazza's authority in physiology is so great that even Darwin's name scarcely encourages an independent opinion. Let us consider the facts.

When we see horses, dogs, or men tremble from fear in the height of summer, at a temperature of 37°, and under the burning rays of the sun, one is inclined to think it is not from any necessity of warming themselves, all the more because monkeys, elephants, and many other animals always found at the equator tremble when they are frightened, even in their tropical countries.

In fever our teeth chatter while the temperature of the body is over 40°, and human economy, far from seeking to heat the blood by trembling, seems rather to stand in need of some mechanism which would cool it, so as to preserve life. After severe exertion or protracted work with the arms, our hands tremble, even when we are panting with heat. When exhausted after the forced marches which I had to make during my studies of fatigue, I have noticed that in the evening, on my return from the peak of Monte Viso or from the highest glaciers of Monte Rosa, my legs trembled, although the temperature of my body was one or two degrees above the normal. Tea, alcohol, coffee, and many stimulating medicines cause a very visible tremor. In convulsive laughter, pleasure, intoxication, voluptuous enjoyment, anger, when the necessity for heating the blood is certainly not apparent, one trembles also, the voice vibrates and the legs shake. All this makes it probable that Darwin is right, and more decidedly do I incline to his side when I think of the disastrous effects which trembling produces during fear. Seals and many animals, of which I shall speak more in detail in the chapter on Fright, tremble so violently that they cannot make their escape, and allow themselves to be overcome and miserably killed. How can we, amongst the sublime perfections which we admire in organisms, admit the contradiction that an animal, in order to warm itself, does not flee from danger but trembles till it is killed, whereas in running away, it could warm itself much better and

---

[16] Darwin, chap. iii., p. 67.

[17] Mantegazza, chap. vii., p. 119.

save its life as well? But the question must not be judged in this way. The divergent opinions which arise in the interpretation of facts are most difficult to resolve in science, because to one of the adversaries there always remains a certain territory in which he may intrench himself.

III

In order to learn the actual nature of trembling we must first see how the muscles are made and how they act.

If we look at a muscular filament as fine as a hair under the microscope, we see that it consists of nearly a hundred extremely fine fibrillæ lying close to each other in the form of bundles. It is these which together form those minute threads seen with the naked eye in fibrous meat. Each fibril, seen under a powerful microscope magnifying three or four hundred times, appears formed of a series of muscular elements, or, let us say, of so many little boxes, piled one on the top of the other like a battery and about two-thousandths of a millimetre in thickness. Each little box is prismatic in form and terminates in two flat ends. It was an English physiologist who described these little boxes for the first time; they are therefore known in science as Bowman's muscular elements. The resemblance of each fibril to a voltaic pile is so great that some have tried, but in vain, to establish an analogy between their functions.

The nerves which go to the muscles send their branches to every fibre, like the fine cords of a match which serve the purpose of firing the powder in the mines at a distance, or, to make use of another simile nearer the truth, although still very far from reality, like the thin wire which conducts the electric spark to a cartouch of dynamite. When the nerve discharges its influence into the muscles, a very rapid molecular change takes place in the substance contained in the cartouches or muscular boxes, which contract, pressing their ends close together. Scarcely has the action of the nerves ceased than they relax and resume their previous form. It is well known, that when a muscle contracts, it becomes thicker and shorter; it suffices to take hold of the arm a little above the elbow and then to bend it in order to feel how the biceps muscle swells and hardens. Wherever a muscular contraction is produced, we may always imagine it as the transverse thickening of an innumerable series of little prismatic boxes, which at the same time shorten in the direction of the fibres.

The blood, which circulates in all the most remote corners of the organism, brings, so to speak, fresh explosive materials to charge the muscles again, cleansing it also from the soot and scoriæ. The movement of the blood in the cells and fibres of the body is like a brook flowing through a village, from which every house may draw water for its needs, and into which any useless articles may be thrown and so carried away.

If we stop our ears with our fingers, we hear a dull noise, like the distant roar of cannon or a prolonged peal of thunder. This thunder is produced by the contraction of the muscles, for the nerves do not exercise a constant action on the fibres, but develop their influence in very rapid, irregular shocks, like the rattle of musketry in a battle.

It is seldom that a nervous discharge takes place all at once, like a volley of shot, in order to produce an instantaneous contraction, or, as physicians would say, a clonic contraction. Generally the discharges in muscular exertion begin in a few fibres; when these become weak, others come to reinforce the contraction; these cease, and others are charged; those are exhausted and others take up their work; thus a continuous tension of the muscle may be maintained. We must, therefore, consider the contraction of a muscle as an extremely rapid trembling of its most minute parts. When we become weaker through illness or from any other cause, we tremble because the contractions are so drawn out and distended as to show the elements composing them. If we poison a frog with some substance which diminishes the vitality of the nerves, there is a trembling of the legs at every exertion which the animal makes to move. In the violent and fatal contractions of tetanus, one can hear the muscular noise even at a distance. Those poor dogs which we see in the street cruelly poisoned with strychnine send forth during their convulsions, if laid on a sounding-board, a characteristic sound which arises from the extremely rapid vibrations of their muscles. It is the sound of tetanus.

IV

Trembling may be produced by two opposite causes, either by an excessive development of nervous tension, or by weakness. 'Les tremblements ont deux diverses causes: l'une est qu'il vient quelquefois trop peu d'esprits du cerveau dans les nerfs, et l'autre qu'il y en vient quelquefois trop.' Descartes told us this two hundred years ago.

If we bend the forearm forcibly against the upper arm, as though to touch the shoulder with the clenched fist, we notice at once that our hand trembles, because the discharges, by means of which the contractions are produced and regulated, do not exactly answer their purpose. If we press the butt of the musket too firmly against our shoulder, or shoot with a heavy gun, we hit the mark less easily because of the trembling of our arms. We may, however, in a great measure correct these physiological imperfections; thus it is that a few months of practice in drawing will enable anyone to draw straight lines and to outline with a firm touch.

In order to understand the whole mechanism of trembling, we must remember that in grasping an object, we not only make use of those muscles which bend the fingers but also of those which serve to open the hand. The work of the muscles which oppose a movement, and which are therefore called antagonistic, is extremely efficacious, and is indeed indispensable in order to graduate and regulate muscular actions with accuracy. When we wish to move our eyes, all the muscles enter into tension, but one prevails and guides them to the desired point. When we take hold of the pen to write, we do not only bend the flexors of the fingers but also involuntarily contract the extensors. Without this it would be impossible suddenly to arrest the hand, the eyes, or any other part of the body in rapid motion.

Exhaustion or over-excitement of the nerve-centres destroys the harmony of aim of muscular contractions. The hand trembles, because the tension of the flexors and extensors is no longer evenly and firmly, but jerkily maintained. If we endeavour to keep the arm stretched out, we find we are not able to regulate the nervous discharges in such a manner as to preserve the equilibrium of the muscles during work, they relax and contract alternately on one side or the other; scarcely do the flexors give way, than the antagonist muscles succeed in bending the arm in their direction, then these shorten in their turn, rapidly resuming their previous position; but no sooner has an effort been made by the muscles of the other side, than they are again overcome by the antagonists. In this way a perpetual wavering is brought about, and the organs of the body sway, waver, or tremble according to the rapidity with which the muscles relax, without the will being able to control them.

In joy and intense pain there is a degree of emotion in which the intonation of the voice is changed, because the nerves which move the muscles of the larynx no longer regularly adjust the vocal cords. This is the origin of the *tremolo* which serves to heighten the pathetic expression in singing. Many are scarcely able to speak, but stammer under the influence of an emotion. It is difficult to pitch a loud note and sustain it with expanded chest without the voice trembling; in the same way one cannot scream for any length of time without the voice turning shrill and harsh, because the muscles tire and the movements of the larynx can only be imperfectly regulated; similarly, when we write after running or violent exercise, certain unusual flourishes appear which make the characters unrecognisable.

I have noticed a curious tremor during inspiration in suffering men and animals. I have found it in a less degree also in healthy animals, particularly in dogs. At every inspiration there is a very noticeable tremor of the limbs and of nearly the whole muscular system. The excitement arising in the nerve-centres to produce a contraction of the diaphragm and of the muscles of the thorax seems to have become so strong, that it goes beyond the limits of the respiratory centre and diffuses itself over a great part of the nerves. In anger, fear, and mental perturbations, when the stormy winds of passion rage, waves flow to all parts of the nervous system, then break, revealing themselves in the agitation of the muscles.

Trembling often has a peripheral origin, and may be due to both heat and cold. It is sufficient to hold the arm in water heated up to 48° or 50° in order to produce a visible tremor. This fact, which I observed repeatedly on my brother, corresponds to the chattering of the teeth when a cold stream of air strikes our face.

V

Very excitable dogs often tremble when another dog approaches. I know one that trembles like a leaf whenever, from the height of a second floor, he sees a bigger dog passing in the street. This lively alarm is quite pitiable, and after all most unnecessary, for the most of his supposed rivals do not perceive his presence, nor even look up. But as soon as he catches sight of them in the distance, he becomes suspicious, a feverish shiver goes over him, the hair on his back stands on end, his whole body trembles, while he cowers near the window with ears erect, looking fiercely out of the corners of his eyes, snarling, and showing his teeth—a ridiculous instance of timid arrogance and despised pride.

But most clearly does trembling become manifest during fear. As army surgeon, I had once to be present at the execution of some brigands. It was a summary judgment. A major of the *bersaglieri* put a few questions to one or two, then turning to the captain said simply: 'Shoot them.' Some were dumb-founded and stood open-mouthed, petrified; others seemed indifferent. I remember one lad, of scarcely twenty years of age, who mumbled replies to a few questions, then remained silent, in the position of a man warding off a fatal blow, with lifted arms, extended palms, the neck drawn between the shoulders, the head held sideways, the body bent and drawn backwards. When he heard the dreadful word, he emitted a shrill, heart-rending cry of despair, looked around him, as though eagerly seeking something, then turned to flee and rushed with outspread arms against a wall of the court, writhing, and scratching it as though trying to force an entrance between the stones, like a polype clinging to a rock. After a few screams and contortions, he suddenly sank to the ground, powerless and helpless, like a log. He was pale and trembled as I have never seen anyone tremble since; it seemed as though the muscles had been turned to a jelly which was shaken in all directions.

Even in their minor degrees apprehension and fear make us tremble. When hurried one cannot perform any minute work, the convulsive fingers can grasp nothing. I know timid girls who are ashamed of the trembling of their hands when filling the tea-cups of their guests.

A gentleman in Germany told me some very curious things about his excitability, amongst others that he had had to give up dancing, as his legs left him in the lurch at the least emotion. Everything disturbed his equanimity; if he had to offer his arm to a lady to take her in to dinner, or to walk across the room when in company, the mere thought of being observed made him tremble and totter as though intoxicated.

The kneeling attitude which one finds amongst all people as a sign of adoration, love, and as the position of one imploring pardon or mercy, must be ascribed to the physiological fact that strong emotions cause a sudden trembling of the legs and oblige us to sink to the ground.

VI

In thinking over the question of trembling, memory has become so excited, that wherever I seek a place of repose amongst my recollections, I still see people before me, trembling. The first, dimmest of these recollections is of an old uncle of mine, a veteran, who, while I was a child, used to take me on his knee to tell me about Napoleon's battles, and I would look at his snuff-box shaking in his hands and could not understand why I must help him to steady his fingers, as he showed me the picture of the emperor on his medal. And behind him I see a simple, affectionate old lady who used to say tender words to me with her trembling voice. She was the godmother of my mother, and was always so indulgent with me when I played near her little work-table, and used to watch me contentedly over her spectacles, waiting till I had drawn the thread through the big-eyed needle, and telling me that her hands no longer obeyed her.

Then the trembling fit which came over me in the Alps when I had wandered through a glacier, risking my life at every step, and it seemed a miracle that I should have escaped the dreadful abyss which was ready to engulf me. Again, amongst the first recollections of my hospital life, I see the emaciated faces of trembling invalids poisoned with quinine or mercury; the convalescent, sitting up in bed, unable to steady the cup in their hand; the anæmic, who, from loss of blood, performed every movement tremblingly; the ravingly hysterical, who only found rest in sleep.

I recall again the times and places when I have hurried excitedly to fires, boiler-explosions, to the ruins of fallen buildings, and have seen men whose teeth chattered in consequence of burns received, strong workmen laid on stretchers who trembled from the effect of their contusions. I remember the night-watches, when we used to relieve each other in attendance on those unfortunate beings who had fallen a prey to tetanus, and whose life had to be prolonged by inhalations of chloroform. In the long, silent halls of the infirmaries I still see the pitiable look of those suffering from *tabes dorsalis* or *paralysis agitans*, who could not stand steadily, nor indeed erect themselves at all, as though a curse were agitating the muscles, over which the will had lost all control, and which at last became so rigid that even the bones of the skeleton were bent and deformed.

But let me turn away from these recollections of misery, now when I see crowding before me more cheerful pictures—of that solemn tremor with which I have seen parents overcome, who, at the wedding of their children, could no longer hold the glass in their hands, and stammered unintelligible words with tears in their eyes. I see young poets, too, who cannot steady the paper as they rise to read their verses to a merry company; and busy housewives with trembling lips, and faces beaming with satisfaction, who have to sit down because they cannot subdue their exultation at their success; and lastly, relatives who, with convulsive hands, embrace each other in the joy of meeting once more.

I have known men so nervous that they had to retire at the slightest emotion, lest they should betray an agitation which seemed ridiculous to them; and I have seen others support themselves with a hand on a table or chair that they might not tremble when they heard a moving speech or saw the representation of a tragedy at the theatre.

I remember onanists who, from fear of their trembling-fits, have been reduced to the humiliation of confessing their loathsome, degrading vice; love-sick friends who have been startled at the trembling of their hands, which altered the character of their writing; colleagues who have consulted me on account of a trembling which appeared after they were exhausted by mental work; and persons who, in consequence of a fright, were subject to trembling for the rest of their lives.

VII

But it is in *delirium tremens* that fear and trembling together form the most awful torture, the most horrible punishment of human nature. During my life as a physician I have only seen three such cases, and the faces of the wretches float before me, covered, as it were, with a veil of profound melancholy.

I shall condense the observations which I made into a single picture, so as not to detain the reader too long amongst such scenes of misery.

Generally, one is called in haste to a patient who is vomiting, or who is thought to be seized with insanity. One finds a wan, emaciated man, who looks at us indifferently, or answers with a few impolite words in a dull, rough voice. Relatives, wife and children, who stand frightened around the bed, tell us that he has been immoderate in drinking, and had been brought home intoxicated the night before; that he had grumbled the whole night long, and did not rise in the morning because of excessive fatigue; that he had felt sick all day and had had no appetite, and that he had then begun to vomit. When he shows his tongue, we see that it is covered with a thick, whitish coat, as in catarrh of the stomach.

In the first period of the illness, the hands do not tremble as they lie on the coverlet, but when the patient tries to take a cup or a spoon, they shake so that everything is upset and spilt. At night the dreams, which have already awakened him in fright, assume the character of a positive hallucination. Often patients spring out of bed, crying that a snake is twining round their neck, and they tear, panting, the clothes from their body, and wander about naked, writhing, as though trying to release their neck from a noose, to free themselves from fetters in which their madness has bound them fast.

Then they grow quiet again, but the delirium has broken out and will develop, leaving them no more peace. They will lend life to every shadow, and see perpetually before them reptiles and insects crawling about and multiplying. What agony! Ever and anon they cry out that monstrous spiders or venomous scorpions are creeping from the walls on to the bed; that black cats with fiery eyes are crouching on their breast; that wolves with open jaws or mad dogs with foaming mouths are biting them, or that loathsome rats, mingling with a black swarm of beetles, are gnawing at their vitals. And then the patients, tortured, annihilated by fear, writhe, gnashing their teeth, groaning, howling, sobbing. They bite their hands, tear the bed-clothes, bury their nails in their faces disfigured with rage. Then they rise to escape, and fall heavily backwards into bed, exhausted, pallid, with distorted face, a rattling in the throat, and their eyes rolling in the most awful despair.

Sometimes this hideous storm blows over, and a little calm returns. The patients are languid, and when questioned answer intelligibly but crossly. In lucid intervals some regret their faults, and say that they drank in order to forget their misfortunes or their misery, but these are only rays of light in the midst of ruins shrouded in darkness. Nearly all remain indifferent to the desolation of the family, shake their heads disconsolately, and talk of suicide. At every feverish attack, by whatever cause produced, the frenzy becomes so great that they must be bound and secured in a strait-jacket.

The trembling increases, the patient cannot sleep; he chatters, walks up and down, wandering about the room like a lost dog. We make out from his laments that the hallucination is gradually taking possession of all his senses. In stammering, disconnected words, he complains from time to time that he is poisoned, has the taste of something loathsome in his mouth, and he rejects everything because he fears treachery. He says there are chemical vapours rising in the room which will suffocate him, and then he runs hither and thither raging, fighting the air with clenched hands, pressing himself close to the wall, or rushing to the window, throwing to the ground furniture and utensils from which he thinks he sees the pestilential vapours poured forth.

My whole life long I shall remember with a shudder the night which, as a student, I spent with one of these unhappy wretches. It was at that time when physicians believed that the danger could be averted and the delirium shortened by a speedy letting of blood. I had been sent by an old physician into a squalid garret, in order to bleed a patient. I found him in bed raging violently. He was a sturdy porter, with inflamed face and swollen neck-veins. When I tried to take him by the arm, he looked at me with bloodshot eyes that seemed to devour me. Then he began to mumble and tremble, pouring forth oaths like stormy thunder, and howling like a lost soul. 'No, no, help! Stop the murderer who is going to kill me—he has a razor to cut my throat!' His face wore a terrible expression of fear, the furrows on the brow, the dilated nostrils, contracted lips, the gnashing of the teeth, gave evidence of a desperate struggle. Then he writhed in our arms, trying to escape, while we held him back. 'Help!' he screamed, 'they are going to throw me out of the window, on to the bayonets below! Help, quick, take those cut-throats away! Do you not see that the street is full of soldiers and executioners, who are climbing up on ladders to stab me?' Until at last, worn out, bathed in perspiration, livid, breathless, still cursing and murmuring, he fell gradually into the lethargy of the dying.

When the disease grows worse, the delirium becomes continual, the trembling increases, the muscles swell to such a degree that it seems as though they would burst. One might almost think that a furious demon were hidden within, agitating the body in the bed, distorting it, hurling it to and fro, as though to shatter it completely. The most terrible apparitions are those of spectres. Some of these are so horrible that the patients are paralysed with dread. They suddenly send forth a terrible shriek, hold their hands in front of them, throw the head back, but still think they see the lean and colourless face of some dead man whom they call by name. Disguised enemies with fleshless countenance, wrapped in grave-clothes, come to lead them away with them; skeletons stride through the room, rattling their bones and gnashing their teeth with devilish glances.

Then Death, dressed in all the horrors of the most corrupt reality, appears to lower them into the grave. 'Take away this rotting corpse which those wretches have put into my bed! Do you not see that it is a liquid, loathsome mass, a putrefied abomination, and that the worms are crawling about the body?' And they hold their nose to exclude the putrid smell, and look at their hands, on which they see clots of blood, livid streaks, and the revolting blackness of gangrene. Sometimes all ends suddenly, but often they sleep after the delirium has lasted three or four days, and on waking, fall into imbecility, die exhausted, or else become quite mad.

CHAPTER IX

THE EXPRESSION OF THE FACE

I

The eye examines the human countenance with such rapidity and such accuracy that no one will ever succeed in giving in words a picture of the minute details and fugitive traits which we see appear and disappear on the face during emotion. Even the greatest masters were not very exact in such-like descriptions, and had recourse to similes, to flowery and metaphorical language. If, for instance, we write that someone looked at us in astonishment or fear, we indicate an endless series of gradations of the same feeling, differing one and all from each other in intensity and effect, and we leave it to the judgment of the reader to choose that which seems to him best suited to the instance, without our having the means to demonstrate it to him. When we say to a friend, 'I must give you a piece of bad news,' there appears a sudden change in his face, his look and his gestures, which touches us. But there is no art of words capable of describing it, because we cannot measure the imperceptible changes which take place in the movement of the eyes, the widening of the pupils, the colouring of the cheeks, the trembling of the lips, the dilatation of the nostrils, the acceleration of the breath, the gestures of the hands, the attitude of the head and trunk.

Certain fine characteristic traits of the face disappear under the magnifying glass like the diamond burning away in the crucible. The aspect of the countenance is impalpable; its beauties are covered by a subtile, delicate veil, which we cannot touch without tearing it and destroying the charm.

It is on this account that I stretch out my hand hesitatingly to take hold of the scalpel and lay bare the head of a corpse, in order to cut through the skin and detach the muscles. When I have separated the muscles of the face from the bones of the skull, a mask like a funnel of flesh remains in my hand. Oh, how ugly is the human face seen from the wrong side! We do not recognise ourselves; we cannot believe that this fibrous web and muscular network represent the most beautiful and expressive part of the organism; that this is the face formerly so graceful in its movements and play of feature, so inexhaustible in its expressions of benevolence and affection. It is a thorough disillusion, a sad sight, as when one sees the framework and the burnt-out rockets of fireworks in broad daylight, or when, at the end of the play, we examine near-to the daubs and rags of a dazzling theatrical decoration. We cannot believe that it is this fibrous flesh which lends us the aspect, the characteristic traits, the expression of our ego; that it is on this thin leaf of muscle that each writes his life-story; that it is the chance arrangement of these parts which impels us to mysterious sympathies, to indifference, antipathy, repugnance; that it is the unfathomable secret of these organs which unconsciously draws men together or apart, like atoms that meet, separate, or remain indissolubly united.

II

Leonardo da Vinci, who was certainly one of the greatest connoisseurs of the human countenance, had studied its anatomy with such ardour that the drawings of his preparations still excite the admiration of the learned by the accuracy of the most minute details.

'*First study Science, and then follow her daughter Art*', said Leonardo to his pupils; and these words are worthy of him who was not only a great artist and mathematician, and an illustrious philosopher, but who earned the title, far more difficult to acquire, of being an innovator in science, and one of the founders of the experimental method.

We must not begin the study of the face with that of the human anatomy. The web of muscles is so close, the direction of the fibres so intricate, that we are baffled unless we know the origin of these muscles in the lower animals, unless we investigate their office in simpler beings, and the modifications which they undergo on the zoological ladder.

The most important parts of the face are the apertures of the mouth and nostrils. These alone never disappear, however the form of the head may alter in different animals. The lips, nose, and chin may become unrecognisable, as in birds; the eye may become a mere point, as in the mole, or may disappear altogether as in certain animals living in caves; but the mouth always remains, because the alimentary canal is the most useful organ of the body. It appears even in animals that have neither heart nor lungs, and is formed like a funnel at its upper end. It is this end of the alimentary canal which we call the face. However grotesque such a mode of expression may seem, it is yet the expression of truth.

The development of the facial muscles is proportioned to the need of seizing prey and crushing the food. In frogs, fish, reptiles, birds, that swallow their food whole, one may say that the face is wanting; they have no expression except in the eye. In birds, the functions of the facial nerve are restricted to a little filament distributed to the cutaneous muscles of the neck, which produces that ruffling of the feathers and erection of the crest which is the characteristic expression of their feelings. The more complex the movements of seizing and devouring the prey become, the more complicated becomes the formation of the mouth. The lips must be mobile in order to suck the nipple of the breast, in the manner of a cupping-glass. Later, they serve to bring the fragments which must be masticated between the jaws, and further, they must be capable of being drawn upwards, as in the dog when he shows his teeth in preparing to bite.[18]

---

[18] Darwin believed that animals show their teeth in order to let their weapons be seen, and in this way to be more feared. This explanation does not seem to me quite exact, as animals are obliged to raise the lips when

Then come the movements of the jaws furnished with fangs for tearing, crushing, breaking, gnawing, and again the very complex movements of the tongue in drinking, licking, collecting the food in the mouth, forming it into a bolus, and finally despatching it.

Of all animals, monkeys possess the greatest development of the facial muscles. This is owing principally to the circumstance that they eat everything, being half carnivorous, half herbivorous, and make use of the mouth as an organ for seizing the prey, and assisting the hands in tearing, skinning, and continually preparing the food.

The countenance of the monkey is of unexampled mobility; in a few minutes one sees all expressions pass over it, from desire to contempt, from cunning to innocence, from attention to carelessness, from love to rage, from aggression to fear, from joy to sadness.

III

One of the reasons why the facial muscles move more easily, is their diminutive size. It was Spencer who first clearly developed this idea, and I know of nothing more fundamental in the language of the emotions. 'Supposing,' he says, 'a feeble wave of nervous excitement to be propagated uniformly throughout the nervous system, the part of it discharged on the muscles will show its effects most where the amount of inertia to be overcome is least. Muscles which are large, and which can show states of contraction into which they are thrown only by moving limbs or other heavy masses, will yield no signs; while small muscles, and those which can move without overcoming great resistances, will visibly respond to this feeble wave. Hence must result a certain general order in the excitation of the muscles, serving to mark the strength of the nervous discharge and of the feeling accompanying it.... It is because the muscles of the face are relatively small, and are attached to easily moved parts, that the face is so good an index of the amount of feeling.'[19]

This law, however, is in my opinion insufficient to explain the expressions of the face, because we have very fine, small muscles in the ear, the skin, and elsewhere, that yet take no part in the expression, although the resistance they offer is very small.

Great importance must, I think, be attached to the continual use of certain muscles, and to the different excitability of their nerves. The muscles which we most frequently put into movement are also those which most easily betray the excitement of the nerve-centres. It is so with the ear of the horse and dog, which is a faithful mirror of everything they feel, of all their emotions; while the ears of man, although possessing the same muscles, remain immovable even during the strongest emotion, and solely because we never make use of them.

---

they bite, so that the soft parts of the mouth covering the jaws may not be injured. It suffices to watch a dog in order to convince oneself that the showing of the teeth must be an act preparatory to that of biting.

[19] *Principles of Psychology*, vol. ii., pp. 542-43.

The facial muscles are agitated by every little shock which the nervous system receives, because they are already perpetually in movement in respiration, speaking, chewing, and in the defence and use of the organs of sense situated in the head. We very often meet people who, in consequence of increased irritability of the nerve-centres, suffer from nervous contractions of the face, which make them wink rapidly, contort the mouth and frown, but we never notice similar disturbances in hands or feet, or in any other part of the body.

The varying resistance which the different nerves of the organism oppose to the nervous currents is an important factor in expression. The proximity of the muscles of the face, and especially of the eyes, to the brain renders the nervous discharges easier. Death always begins in the parts furthest removed from the centre, the legs grow rigid sooner than the arms, and the eye is the last to be extinguished.

The subject at present under consideration is a field of study which physiologists have perhaps too much neglected. Johannes Müller,[20] the father of modern physiology, in speaking of those 'movements which depend upon mental conditions,' expresses himself in the following manner: 'The extremely varied expression of the lineaments of the face in different passions, shows that, according to the various states of the mind, entirely different groups of fibres of the facial nerve are brought into activity. The reasons of this phenomenon, of these relations of the facial muscles to special passions, are totally unknown.'

Wishing to make a few experiments on the facial nerve, to see whether I should succeed in discovering anything in this obscure field of physiology, I laid bare the facial nerve, at its point of departure from the skull, in a dog rendered insensible with chloral, and then fixed two electrodes in such a manner that I was sure of being able to irritate the whole nerve by means of an electric current. While using irritants so weak that they were imperceptible on the tongue, I observed that they could cause a contraction of the muscles of the forehead and make the ears move, while the whole muzzle remained still as in an animal in an attentive attitude. When I used a slightly stronger stimulus, the muscles of the nose and eyelids and the zygomatic muscle moved; when the irritant was still more intensified, the muscles of the under-lip contracted and the mouth opened; while under very strong irritations, the dog assumed the fierce expression of one about to attack.

There is something fantastic in those experiments on decapitated animals of which the brain has been destroyed, and the face of which may be taken up in the hand like a mask of flesh. While applying an electric current to the motor nerves, one sees the features reanimate themselves, and a series of expressions pass over them one after another—attention, joy, rage, as though the electric apparatus applied to the facial nerve represented the commands of the brain or psychic impressions which in reality no longer exist.

---

[20] J. Müller: *Handbuch der Physiologie des Menschen*, 1840, ii. 92.

The mechanical part of expression is, therefore, much simpler than one thinks. When a psychic operation takes place in the nerve-centres, the tension propagates itself along the nervous lines of least resistance. The more sensitive we are, the more graceful, beautiful, expressive, and fascinating is the curving of the lips produced by a smile. Peasants and coarse, dull persons cannot smile, with them the stimulus increases until it bursts out in a noisy, vacant laugh.

The nerve-paths are constructed in such a way that the brain does not need trouble itself about the muscular movements. It is the intensity of the excitement which produces the expression; the stronger it is, the more numerous are the paths through which the nervous tension forces its way; as it increases, it overcomes all obstacles and resistance confronting it in other paths impassable till that movement, and contracts muscles which till then had remained neutral.

The effects of the passions are reflected principally in the muscles of the face and respiration. No other function has to adapt itself more continuously than this last to the needs of the organism, standing as it does in close connection with all changes taking place in the nerve-centres. The muscles most vividly expressing passion are nearly all respiratory muscles.

IV

Our nervous system is so constituted that during violent emotion its activity discharges itself in all directions, and herein must we seek the reason of the resemblance between such different conditions as laughter and weeping, pain and pleasure.

It is the quantity, not the quality, of the stimulus which has weight on the scale of the expressions. This statement of mine will appear clearer if we study the phenomena produced by tickling.

When monkeys are touched in the arm-pit they twist and writhe, laugh, and emit sounds like human cries. The nerve-centres are very susceptible to the mechanical excitation of certain nerves, to contacts which fill us with the most pleasant and delicious sensations, or burst like a storm upon the organism.

We have heard of persons who let themselves be tickled to death, and there are many sensitive natures that can scarcely bear the most ardent enjoyments of life.

Here are prayers for pity, unconscious denials, entreaties in tearful tones, exclamations of astonishment, humble or clamorous voices, cries of joy or unsuppressed sighs, lamentations as of those who suffer, moans with which human nature seems to succumb.

Voluptuous enjoyment causes a vibration of the nerves, and forces from our lips the same moans as pain, which dulls the fire of life.

The respiratory movements are accelerated and panting, sometimes arrested, then recommencing irregularly; the breath pours stormily from the dilated nostrils, there is a singing in the ears, the heart beats more rapidly, and its pulsations resound with such violence that we wonder how a slight tickling of the nerves can produce such inward agitation.

The vital centres are stunned by a mysterious emotion—by a charm which deadens the senses and slackens the reins of control. With the cessation of the moderating force of the brain, the harmony of aim is destroyed, oppression seizes us, and words almost unconsciously spoken are now interrupted and repeated, anon breathless and drawn out, and are at last extinguished in the languor of a swoon. The dim eyes look upwards or hide moodily behind their lids, roll frightened in their orbits, or fill with tears of joy and close with the uncertain glance of the dying. The arms move convulsively, wildly, clutching, grasping, writhing. The teeth gnash and show themselves; there is a moaning and howling as though in man the animal soul had reawakened.

And at last, when the storm is past, the convulsions and trembling die away gradually like the flashes of lightning that follow the roar of retreating thunder. But the languid glance, the flaccid features, the moisture of the skin, the fatigue of the limbs, the spasmodic contractions of the muscles, the quivering of the voice, the thirst, the palpitation, the weakness, the lethargy of the senses, remain like the traces of a morbid paroxysm, like the depression after a great misfortune.

CHAPTER X

THE EXPRESSION OF THE FOREHEAD AND EYE

I

Those who have not carefully followed the history of scientific progress think that the theory of evolution is solely Darwin's work. The same thing has happened as after a victory, when public opinion lauds the name of a single general, whereas the action of others was no less efficacious and decisive in winning the battle. But in this case it would be an injustice not to award the greatest praise to Herbert Spencer, whom Darwin himself called '*the great expounder*' of the principle of evolution. So soon as 1855, in the first edition of his 'Principles of Psychology,' Spencer maintains the doctrine of evolution, when, as he says, it was 'ridiculed in the world at large and frowned upon in the scientific world.'

In the second edition of his 'Principles of Psychology,' Spencer added a chapter entitled, 'The Language of the Emotions,' which is of great value to us, as it was printed a few months before Darwin published his book, 'The Expression of the Emotions.'

One of the most important ideas, physiologically speaking, which Spencer has formulated is the following: 'The molecular motion disengaged in any nerve-centre by any stimulus, tends ever to flow along lines of least resistance throughout the nervous system, exciting other nerve-centres, and setting up other discharges. The feelings of all orders, moderate as well as strong, which from instant to instant arise in consciousness, are the correlatives of nerve-waves continually being generated and continually reverberating throughout the nervous system—the perpetual nervous discharge constituted by these perpetually-generated waves, affecting both the viscera and the muscles, voluntary and involuntary.'

The ideas developed by Darwin on the origin of the expressions have such a striking resemblance, even identity, with Spencer's doctrine, that Darwin felt himself obliged to make the following declaration in a foot-note: 'I may state, in order that I may not be accused of trespassing on Mr. Spencer's domain, that I announced in my "Descent of Man" that I had then written a part of the present volume.'[21]

The origin of the movements of expression, as propounded by Spencer and more amply developed by Darwin in his book, does not convince me. The profound admiration which I cherish for these two great masters has made me timid in deviating from their path, but since the facts which presented themselves to me during my studies have convinced me that the same results might be obtained in another way, it

---

[21] Ch. Darwin: *The Expression of the Emotions.* London, 1872, p. 10.

is my duty to communicate those observations and experiments which point to another solution of the problem.

I shall here quote a passage from Spencer's 'Language of the Emotions,' thus drawing, as we say, from the well of the great philosopher himself.

'Throughout the animal kingdom, non-pleasurable feelings are most frequently and most variously excited during antagonism. Among inferior types of creatures antagonism habitually implies combat, with all its struggles and pains. Though in man there are many sources of non-pleasurable feelings other than antagonism, and though antagonism itself ends in combat only when it rises to an extreme, yet as among inferior ancestral types antagonism is the commonest and most conspicuous accompaniment of non-pleasurable feeling, and continues to be very generally an accompaniment in the human race, there is organically established a relation between non-pleasurable feeling and the muscular actions which antagonism habitually causes. Hence those external concomitants of non-pleasurable feeling which constitute what we call its expression, result from incipient muscular contractions of the kinds accompanying actual combat.

'But how does this explain the first and most general mark of non-pleasurable feeling—a frown? What have antagonism and combat to do with that corrugation of the brow which, when slight, may indicate a trifling ache or a small vexation, and when decided, may have for its cause bodily agony, or extreme grief, or violent anger? The reply is not obvious, and yet, when found, is satisfactory.

'If you want to see a distant object in bright sunshine, you are aided by putting your hand above your eyes; and in the tropics, this shading of the eyes to gain distinctness of vision is far more needful than here. In the absence of shade yielded by the hand or by a hat, the effort to see clearly in broad sunshine is always accompanied by a contraction of those muscles of the forehead which cause the eyebrows to be lowered and protruded; so making them serve as much as possible the same purpose that the hand serves.... Now if we bear in mind that during the combats of superior animals, which have various movements of attack and defence, success largely depends on quickness and clearness of vision ... it will be manifest that a slight improvement of vision, obtained by keeping the sun's rays out of the eyes, may often be of great importance, and where the combatants are nearly equal, may determine the victory.... Hence, we may infer that during the evolution of those types from which man more immediately inherits, it must have happened that individuals in whom the nervous discharge accompanying the excitement of combat, caused an unusual contraction of these corrugating muscles of the forehead, would, other things equal, be the more likely to conquer and to leave posterity—survival of the fittest tending in their posterity to establish and increase this peculiarity.'

If this interpretation of Spencer, which Darwin expanded, were true, the consequences would be, that in the long succession of generations animals would have gradually rid themselves of that which is injurious and fatal to them. But this law does not verify itself in the least, rather do we see, in studying violent emotions, that the more serious the danger the greater is the predominance both in number and strength of injurious phenomena. We have already seen that trembling and cataplexy render us unable to flee or defend ourselves, and we shall now be convinced that in critical moments we see less distinctly than when we are tranquil.

In the face of these facts we must admit that not all phenomena of fear can be explained by the theory of selection. In their extreme degrees they are morbid phenomena indicating an imperfection of the organism. One might almost say that nature had not been able to find a substance for brain and spinal cord which should be extremely sensitive, and yet should never, under the influence of exceptionally strong stimuli, exceed in its reaction those physiological limits which are best adapted to the preservation of the animal.

But before we go further, let us consider those facts which seem to contradict the hypothesis of Spencer and Darwin.

II

We all know that the pupil through which the rays of light pass, in order to reach the posterior part of the eye, dilates and contracts with great facility. In the cat its form is variable; generally elliptic, it becomes in a strong light very narrow and nearly shut, appearing like a slit scarcely wider than a hair; towards evening, or in a dark place during the day, it dilates in such a manner that the iris nearly disappears, and one can see the greenish, phosphorescent background of the eye.

The iris is like a circular curtain which closes in a strong light and opens in the dark, regulating automatically the amount of light necessary for sight without causing injury to the eye.

The perfection of our machine is such, that some indispensable mechanisms not only work automatically, without any participation of the will or consciousness, but often also without needing either spinal cord or brain, as those few nerve-cells, found in the organs in the form of microscopic ganglia, suffice for the reflex movements. This harmony by which the body assures the performance of its most important functions, by putting in motion several mechanisms at the same time, all of which are directed to the same end, is worthy of meditation.

The mechanism of these movements of the iris is very complicated; I have noticed that whenever the vessels dilate, the pupil contracts, and when the vessels contract, the pupil dilates.[22]

This relation between the blood-vessels of the iris and its movements has many important advantages; as, for instance, during sleep, when the vessels dilate, the pupil contracts, thus preventing the light from being felt too vividly. In inflammation of the eye, light exercises an irritating and injurious influence; but the vessels during

---

[22] A. Mosso: *Sui movimenti idraulici dell' iride.* R. Accademia di Torino, 1875.

inflammation are always dilated, the pupil is therefore narrower, and the light which strikes the back of the eye less intense, recovery being consequently more speedy.

After copious loss of blood, in fatigue, deep depression, in pain, and similar cases, the vessels contract and the pupil dilates, in this way allowing many things to be seen which would be imperceptible for want of light if the pupil were contracted.

All this seems perfect as an apparatus, but unfortunately it has grave defects.

Our eye is like a photographic machine, and the pupil acts like the diaphragm which photographers put before the lens, for in our eye, too, there is a lens similar to that of the photographic camera, behind the diaphragm of the iris. When there is little light, the photographer puts in a diaphragm with a wider opening, but then the picture becomes dull, because the rays of light in passing further from the centre of the lens and on its peripheral edge produce a picture with indistinct outlines. Photographers, therefore, in order to obtain a picture clear in all its parts, prefer a very strong light, and make use of a diaphragm with a very small opening. These are also the best conditions for distinct vision; for if we observe the eyes of a person who is looking into distance, or is absent-minded, and then hold a small object before him, we see that the pupil immediately contracts.

But this wonderfully perfect mechanism ceases to act as soon as the animal or the man is subjected to violent emotion. When the vessels contract during fear or a struggle, or in any other exertion, the pupil immediately dilates, and the picture loses in distinctness. If we watch fighting dogs, cats, or men, we at once perceive that the eye has become blacker, and that the pupil is at its maximum dilatation.

But how shall we explain, by means of the hypothesis of Spencer and Darwin, the fact that nocturnal animals present with equal precision the same movements in the expression of the forehead and eyes? Why, for the sake of such a small advantage as being able to see a little better when we have the light in our eyes, is there such a complicated muscular apparatus always in operation, while nature has not provided against a far more serious defect, as is the confusion of images caused by the too great dilatation of the iris?

In order to appreciate the extent of the defect of vision during emotion, I made the following experiment, together with Dr. Falchi. We took a small sample of writing from Snell's tables, and then determined what was the greatest distance at which it could be easily read by a certain person; then, on some pretext, we scolded or reproached the subject in such a manner as to occasion a sudden and strong emotion. When we then requested the same person to read the writing, he was no longer able to do so at the same distance, but had to approach the tablet, often by a few steps, in order to see as before. A violent muscular exertion, a few turns on the trapeze or in the gymnastic rings, a race, the rapid ascent of a staircase, also diminish the acuteness of vision in a noticeable manner.

III

When one considers as a whole the symptoms by which fear reveals itself, one might almost think that it was a product of heredity and selection. Animals that are easily frightened, a disciple of Darwin would say, are those which can more easily avoid danger and save themselves; these produce young, and perpetuate their timidity in their posterity. But we know that the phenomena of fear are the morbid exaggeration of physiological facts. Animals cannot become continually more timorous by means of hereditary transmission; the necessity of struggling brings other faculties than those of flight and fear into play, and effect the preservation of the species in another way. Our organism is not such a perfect machine as to be able to resist or adapt itself to all conditions of environment; there are inevitable necessities against which selection is of no avail.

In my opinion, although we may accept the principle of Spencer and Darwin as an explanation of many things, we yet cannot extend it to all phenomena. Spencer and Darwin were not physiologists enough; in their studies of the emotions they did not sufficiently seek the causes of the phenomena observed by them in the functions of the organism. There are, so to speak, hierarchies in the parts composing our machine, for all functions are not equally important. But in the whole of the vital economy one notices the preponderance and supremacy of the blood-vessels. It is so indispensable that the organism should profit by all the material procurable for the nutrition of the nerve-centres, that the circulation of the blood in all parts (therefore in the eye also) is subordinated to this prime object.

In this way it seems to me the fact may be explained that the blood-vessels of the iris contract during strong emotions, notwithstanding that this produces excessive dilatation of the pupil, and that the back of the eye becomes anæmic, although this contraction of the vessels of the retina is disadvantageous to distinct vision.

We often hear persons, speaking of some great fright, say: 'I was like one struck blind, I could see nothing.' Travellers tell of serpents blind with fear, that bit the shadows and branches of the trees, blunting their teeth and shedding their poison fruitlessly.

Darwin maintains that there are two distinct causes for the frown which every little difficulty in a train of thought produces. One is very similar to that propounded by Spencer, of which we have already spoken; the other runs as follows: 'The earliest and almost sole expression seen during the first days of infancy, and then often exhibited, is that displayed during the act of screaming; and screaming is excited, both at first and for some time afterwards, by every distressing or displeasing sensation and emotion,—by hunger, pain, anger, jealousy, fear, &c. At such times the muscles round the eyes are strongly contracted; and this, as I believe, explains to a large extent the act of frowning during the remainder of our lives.[23]

This explanation does not seem to me satisfactory, because it only pushes the question further back, and we must still ask: But why does the child frown when it cries? But, indeed, it suffices to render Darwin's hypothesis improbable, if we call to mind that new-born children frown before they shed a single tear.

The following is the explanation which I offer of this phenomenon.

When we look intently at an object, we must contract all internal and external muscles of the eye. This is indispensable in order to effect the adjustment by which we modify the curvature of the lens in the interior of the eye; that is to say, we alter the lens according to the distance, in the same way as anyone looking through a telescope adjusts it by lengthening or shortening the tube. We have already seen that the pupil must contract when we contemplate an object close to us; thus we cannot direct our gaze towards our nose without a contraction of the pupil.

The most important movement of the external muscles of the eye is that by means of which we produce a convergence of the visual rays from both eyes on the object of attention. Thus, whereas the two eyes are parallel when we are absent-minded or gazing into distance, they converge when fixed on an object near us, as the hands would meet in order to take hold of it. All these movements are effected by a single nerve, called the motor-oculi, between which and the facial nerve there is a certain sympathy, as may be seen in the unconscious movement of the eyelids and forehead when we exercise the eye. And *vice versa*, when we close the lids, we move the eyeball without intending to do so. We may convince ourselves of this if we hold one eye shut with a finger and then close the lid of the other; immediately we feel the eyeball under the finger turn downwards.

The muscles of the eye contract also when we exert ourselves; for instance, if we try by night to look at a small distant light, at the same time lifting a heavy weight, or exerting ourselves in some other way, we see the light double, owing to the involuntary convergence of the eyes. I have photographed several persons during physical exertion, and many of them have quite the appearance of suffering, so pronounced is the contraction of the muscles of the forehead, although it was quite unnecessary. The arrangements of our organism are such that the energy, the tension of the nervous system diffuses itself in various directions, without the possibility, in certain cases, of restricting its influence to limited muscular groups. Thus, if we try to move the ear, the muscles which raise the corner of the mouth also contract; if we merely tell someone to close his eyes, we see the other facial muscles move, often causing involuntary grimaces. Again, we cannot move one eye to the right and the other to the left. Very few can turn the pupil upwards without raising the eyelids, or move the eyebrows separately. All this is due to the difficulty of localising the action of

[23] Ch. Darwin: *The Expression of the Emotions*, p. 225.

the will in the nervous fibres leading only to certain muscles; several groups of fibres seem always drawn simultaneously into the sphere of action, except when there has been much practice in discerning and selecting the fibres which shall accomplish an isolated movement, or when an intentional effort is made, which, however, is a matter of much difficulty.

When animals look attentively at some object, they turn their ears towards it. This movement, which they make in order to collect the sounds, must be preceded by a contraction of the muscles of the forehead and of those serving to turn the auricle of the ear. It is very probable that these movements, noticeable also in monkeys, have been preserved in man, although in attention he no longer moves the ears but only the muscles of the forehead.

In our nature psychic processes are so closely connected with their external sensory manifestations that it is impossible to check the manifestation of nervous activity in the muscles whenever the ideas appear to which these external movements stand in a permanent relation, even when this external communication is quite unnecessary. Thus we see that a man lost in thought gesticulates, making a hundred involuntary movements, and sometimes speaks, although no one is with him to whom he need communicate his ideas. And so it happens that we reproduce the characteristic movements of attention in forehead and eye whenever, in the various contingencies of life or in the development of ideas, an obstacle hinders the progress of thought. As soon as we begin any work which demands greater force of attention and reflection, we immediately and involuntarily put into action the mechanism of forehead and eye, which has always been made use of in intently scrutinising objects.

IV

All will have noticed that when we look intently at anything, all other objects become the more indistinct the further they are removed from the point of attention. This is because we have only one point in our eye in which vision reaches a maximum of acuteness. This point is called the *fovea centralis*, because it looks like a little dimple or funnel of two-tenths of a millimetre in diameter. If the image of an object falls at a distance of only a few millimetres from the *fovea centralis*, the eye can no longer accurately distinguish the colours. Red and green give an impression of palish yellow, violet appears blue. A little further distant, yellow and blue disappear completely, and only light and dark are perceived. This anatomical disposition of the elements destined to perceive the image and colour of objects obliges us to move the eye and bring it into relation with all parts of an object if we wish to examine it minutely. On this account no organ has such precise movements as the eye. If we look at our eye in a mirror, and move our head up and down, to the right and to the left, we see to our astonishment that the eye can remain fixed and motionless. Let the reader repeat this experiment in order to conceive the facility and precision with which the eye fixes on one point which we wish to look at attentively. The restlessness of the eye contemplating an unknown figure, the agitation which is visible in a man when he is afraid of another, and therefore examines him from head to foot in order to be ready to defend himself, or escape an impending danger, is an inevitable consequence of the structure of the eye, which cannot contemplate and embrace a wide field without moving.

When the object is not small enough to be embraced by the simple movements of the eye in its orbit, we bend and turn the head, or move the trunk to right or left; if that does not suffice, we move the whole body. Actors represent fear by exaggerating the attitude peculiar to one intently observing an object.

These movements are so spontaneous and natural, that it costs an effort to keep head and body still when looking at an object situated on one side of us. A feeling of profound contempt, hatred, or pride is necessary before we can pass close to a man with head stiff and erect.

V

Anyone who studies the parts of a machine can judge of the accuracy of its movements, because the structure of a machine represents its function; the dead organism is, therefore, no less important a field for observation and study to the physiologist than the living organism.

When we see, on opening the skull, that three nerves leave the brain to move the eye, and that six muscles are attached to this little ball weighing on an average seven grammes, we may conclude at once that perhaps no other organ has the same variety, independence, and rapidity of movement.

The eye is indeed unrivalled in the complication of its muscles and the number and variety of its nerves by any other organ except the tongue. This explains why both have their own language, and how they are able, by the infinite variation of their movements, to express every emotion of the mind.

The life of the eye lies entirely in its movement. A well-made glass eye which can follow the movements of the real eye can scarcely be distinguished from the latter when placed in the orbit, but when it remains motionless it gives to the countenance a dreadful, spectral appearance.

I have studied the expression of the eye in those born blind. These poor people, who could not even see dim shadows of objects, nor distinguish night from day, as though a sevenfold bandage covered their eyes, used to play instruments and be happy together, nor would anyone have thought that in them the eye was dead, insensible for ever to light; but it was only its movements which gave it an expression of joy and amiability, which inspired confidence and tenderness.

How eloquent is the eye of a dying friend looking at us for the last time, and seeming to reflect all the sadness of an existence fading while still full of hope and aspirations! The eye does not change for many hours, but when you come back to look at the cold semblance of your friend, and bid him a last farewell, the immovable look, the staring eye of death arrests you on the threshold; in it you read the anguish of pain, the horror of an overwhelming misfortune.

There are also in the pupil of the eye vivid expressions which are almost entirely unknown. It is curious to note in the eye of a dog, when quiet, how the pupil dilates and contracts at every emotion. This cannot arise from his looking at near or distant objects. The iris, like the blood-vessels, reflects every little emotion. We do not know these delicate shades in the language of the emotions, because the analysis of physical facts accompanying the expression of the passions has not yet become sufficiently minute and accurate. Between the maximum dilatation of the pupil, so characteristic of fear, and its greatest contraction in sleep, perfect calm and weariness, is the whole intermediate series of movements in which the passions are revealed. There are little alterations in the diameter of the pupil which pass unnoticed, unless one can look closely at the eye, but, by attentively observing a great number of persons, I have convinced myself that it is possible to read the effects of the passions in the movements of the pupil. When the edge of the iris grows narrower and the middle of the eye blacker and larger, it is a sign that we are agitated by a strong emotion which we try in vain to conceal, because the eye, as the poets say, is the window of the soul, through which we look into the depths of the heart.

CHAPTER XI

THE PHYSIOGNOMY OF PAIN

I

Leonardo da Vinci, in his celebrated treatise on painting, in speaking of the difference between laughing and weeping, says: 'In eyes, mouth, and cheeks there is no difference between one who laughs and one who weeps. They are distinguished from each other only by the position of the eyebrows, which contract during weeping, while in one who laughs they are drawn upwards. He who weeps raises the eyebrows at the inner corners, draws them together, wrinkling the skin above them, and turns the corners of the mouth down, while one who laughs draws the corners of the mouth upwards, and has an open, uncontracted brow.'

With these words da Vinci shows the characteristic expression of the face in laughter and in tears; but the physiologist is not content with what satisfies the artist, he seeks the cause and origin of the phenomena, analyses the reason of the difference and similarity in the expression of laughing and weeping, joy and pain.

The impetus which Herbert Spencer and Charles Darwin gave to the study of human nature was so powerful, the progress made so rapid, and the new horizon so vast, that numerous philosophical and scientific books at once became obsolete; and when we now turn over their leaves, we seem to feel the breath of decay, as though we were groping amid the ruins and dust of edifices that have crumbled for centuries.

The study of nature was much easier for the spiritualists and philosophers of the old school than for us, because with little trouble they found reasons which satisfied them, and in their faith they had a strong bulwark that sheltered them from the uncertainty and doubt which follow us everywhere as we grope deeper and deeper, trying to find out the causes of things.

Duchenne de Boulogne, in his well-known book on the mechanism of human physiology, printed in 1862, still maintains that the facial muscles were created for the expression of the soul.

'Le créateur n'a donc pas eu à se préoccuper ici des besoins de la mécanique; il a pu, selon sa sagesse, ou—que l'on me pardonne cette manière de parler—par une divine fantaisie, mettre en action tel ou tel muscle, un seul ou plusieurs muscles à la fois, lorsqu'il a voulu que les signes caractéristiques des passions, même les plus fugaces, fussent écrits passagèrement sur la face de l'homme. Ce langage de la physionomie une fois créé, il lui a suffi, pour le rendre universel et immuable, de donner à tout être humain la faculté instinctive d'ex primer toujours ses sentiments par la contraction des mêmes muscles.

'Il était certainement possible de doubler le nombre des signes expressifs de la physionomie; il fallait, pour cela, que chaque sentiment ne mît en jeu qu'un seul côté de la face. Mais on sent combien un tel langage eût été disgracieux.'[24]

According to Duchenne de Boulogne all passions have a special muscle at their service, which enters into activity in order to express the feelings of the mind; benevolence, joy, laughter, sadness, attention, reflection, lasciviousness, irony, contempt, fright, cruelty, pain, weeping, appear on the human countenance each through the medium of a muscle possessing the privilege of representing a particular emotion.

Duchenne de Boulogne certainly went rather far with his theory of localisations. He treated the face as Gall did the skull and brain. Classifications of mental faculties are too artificial, being derived from an abstraction based on facts and phenomena neither distinct nor definable. Gall wished to localise, so to speak, the metaphysical and theological faculties of the mind in the different parts of the brain, and invented the phrenology which made him famous. But in none of his writings is there any penetration to the real origin of facts. He let his imagination and, more than all, the force of his own eloquence, carry him away, and his phrenology, then called the science of the future and the reforming doctrine of society, has now fallen into oblivion in spite of the prophecies of his followers.

II

Darwin reduced the principles on which the expression of the emotions depends to the following three:

The principle of serviceable associated habits.

That of antithesis.

That of actions due to the constitution of the nervous system, independently from the first of the will and to a certain extent of habit.

According to Darwin the expression of pain depends essentially on the first and third of these principles. He assumes, indeed, that in all animals, in the series of innumerable generations, intense pain has produced the most violent and diverse movements in order to escape its cause.

As the muscles of the thorax and of the vocal organs are those most habitually used, they were called more particularly into action, and animals began to make sounds, to howl and to screech. Darwin believed that vocal sounds were useful to animals, particularly to the young and to those living in community, because in case of danger the cries serve to call the parents or to warn the other animals. These opinions of Charles Darwin open up a wide field for discussion, but for the present I intend to

---

[24] G. B. Duchenne de Boulogne: *Mécanisme de la Physionomie Humaine* (Paris, 1862), p. 32.

speak only of the expression of the face, so as to confine my subject within reasonable limits.

The movements of the facial muscles depend, according to Darwin, on the constitution of the nervous system. We must remark, however, that Darwin took this idea from Herbert Spencer, who, a few years before Darwin published his book, had written a chapter in his 'Principles of Psychology' entitled 'The Language of the Emotions.' Darwin recognised the priority of Herbert Spencer, and I think it advisable to quote a passage from his book, 'The Expression of the Emotions,' so that the reader may become acquainted with one of the most important pages published on the subject of which we are treating:

'As Mr. Herbert Spencer remarks' (says Darwin on p. 71), 'it may be received as an "unquestionable truth that, at any moment, the existing quantity of liberated nerve-force, which in an inscrutable way produces in us the state we call feeling, *must* expend itself in some direction—*must* generate an equivalent manifestation of force somewhere"; so that, when the cerebro-spinal system is highly excited and nerve-force is liberated in excess, it may be expended in intense sensations, active thought, violent movements, or increased activity of the glands. Mr. Spencer further maintains that an "overflow of nerve-force, undirected by any motive, will manifestly take the most habitual routes; and, if these do not suffice, will next overflow into the less habitual ones." Consequently, the facial and respiratory muscles, which are the most used, will be apt to be first brought into action; then those of the upper extremities, next those of the lower, and, finally, those of the whole body.'

The simplicity of this theory is seductive, but it suffices to subject it to a superficial examination in order to see that it does not quite correspond to the facts. If we find out which are the most habitual routes of nerve-force, and write them down in order one after the other, and then compare them with the movements expressing the passions, we shall see that there is not a perfect correspondence.

It was perhaps for this reason that Herbert Spencer afterwards introduced the idea of the nervous lines of least resistance, in order to explain the greater facility with which certain muscles contract, compared to others. 'The molecular motion' (says Spencer) 'disengaged in any nerve-centre by any stimulus, tends ever to flow along lines of least resistance throughout the nervous system.'

The solution of the problem was thus removed to the domain of experimental physiology. The question now is, whether in reality the muscles most commonly in use are those which have nerves offering less resistance, or whether the nervous excitement hidden in the centres is sufficiently strong to allow the resistance made by the nerves to its passage towards the muscles to be disregarded.

Spencer and Darwin gave no proof of their statements, so that it devolves upon us physiologists to discover experimentally whether the intuition of these great philosophers is correct. Darwin was, as usual, very cautious, and in Chapter III., in which he treats of the general principles of expression, after having mentioned the above theory, says: 'Our present subject is very obscure, but, from its importance, must be discussed at some little length; and it is always advisable to perceive clearly our ignorance.'

III

I made a few experiments in order to see whether in reality, as Spencer assumes, there exists a difference of conductibility amongst the various nervous filaments which move the muscles of the face, and which, as we know, are united into one bundle called the facial nerve. I irritated this nerve at its point of departure from the skull, and near the ear, where it is most easily isolated. There is no need to describe the process of irritating the nerves by electric currents. Galvani began in the last century to produce contractions of the muscles by means of electric currents originated by the contact of two metals; and we all know that the contractions of the legs of some skinned frogs, observed by Galvani in Bologna while he was hanging them on the iron railings in his garden, were the beginning of one of the greatest conquests of science, and one of the discoveries which have exercised the greatest influence on civilisation.

The apparatus made use of to irritate the nerves is an invention of Professor Du Bois-Reymond. Many who are not physicians will yet know the apparatus, which is often used in the cure of diseases by electricity; its greatest advantage consists in the facility with which the intensity of the electrical stimulus may be increased or diminished.

After having produced such a profound sleep in a dog by means of chloral that he was insensible, I tried to irritate the nerve which moves the muscles of the face by a very weak electric current. At first the current was so weak that no effect was visible, but as it was increased, a slight contraction of the cutaneous muscle of the neck appeared, and a little movement at the corner of the mouth. It might perhaps be of use to explain here how, in the muscles situated under the skin of the neck, other facial muscles originate, amongst others the so-called risorial muscle; but in order not to interrupt the relation of this experiment, I shall reserve these remarks till the beginning of the next section. The intensity of the electric current when the slight movement of the mouth appeared was equal to 400 units.

If the current is increased, the movement of the lips becomes more apparent, and when the electric irritation of the *facialis* reaches the intensity of 700, a contraction of the orbicular muscle of the eyelids appears, which closes the eyes. At an intensity of 750 the muscles which elevate the upper lip contract. At 820 the nostrils are dilated and elevated. At 950 the contraction of the lips becomes so pronounced that the dog shows his teeth, and his face assumes an aggressive expression. At 1,250 there is a depression of the corners of the mouth, as though produced by pain and disgust. At 1,500 this expression becomes more intense, and the eye is forcibly shut. If the stimulus is still further intensified, the face assumes the fierce expression of an animal about to attack.

I obtained the same results with the animal soon after death.

These experiments show that Herbert Spencer's hypothesis is correct; but we shall presently see that the matter is exceedingly complicated, and that we must take into account other factors no less important in the expression of the face.

IV

The muscles of the face have certainly not the office, as Duchenne de Boulogne thought, of expressing the passions of the soul. To speak frankly and without sentimentality, pedantry, or conventionality, we must recognise that the most important feature of the face is the mouth, and that the mouth is a funnel of flesh attached to the alimentary canal. Sometimes it only serves to seize the prey and receive the food before sending it to the stomach, as is the case in fishes, reptiles, and birds, in which the face is reduced to a minimum. As the apparatus for mastication becomes more complicated with the appearance of teeth for cutting and crushing the food, and of lips for sucking, drinking, and closing the mouth, the more complicated also does the structure of the face become.

One of the most curious things discovered by anatomists is, that many muscles of the face, of great importance in the expression of the emotions, were originally, that is, in the inferior animals, muscles serving a very different purpose. I shall develop this fact briefly, so that the reader may see how difficulties continually increase the nearer science approaches to the origin of things.

We all know that the hedgehog rolls itself up on the approach of danger, its body having the appearance of a ball covered with bristles. This movement is executed by means of a muscle under the skin which covers nearly the whole body, and which contracts in a similar manner to a bag drawn together by a string. Many other animals are similarly furnished with a fine muscular layer which covers the body. In the mole, for instance, this muscular system is well developed. Amongst domestic animals we may mention the dog, the cat, and the horse, in which, although these layers of cutaneous muscles are less compact, they are still sufficiently developed to be noticeable when they enter into action.

We have all remarked the rapid twitching of the skin by which dogs and horses rid themselves of flies. This movement is due to the rapid contraction of one of these muscles. It is easily proved that this is not in reality their office, for they are well developed in birds, fish, and reptiles that do not need to defend themselves from flies in this way.

In all higher animals the traces of organs exist, which remind us of our kinship with the lower animals. Sometimes these organs retrograde from want of use, at other times they remain in existence but fulfil a very different office, and one always much less useful than the original one. Thus the cutaneous muscles still exist under the skin in many parts of the human body, as an inheritance and a sign transmitted to us by generations of animals that have preceded us on the earth.

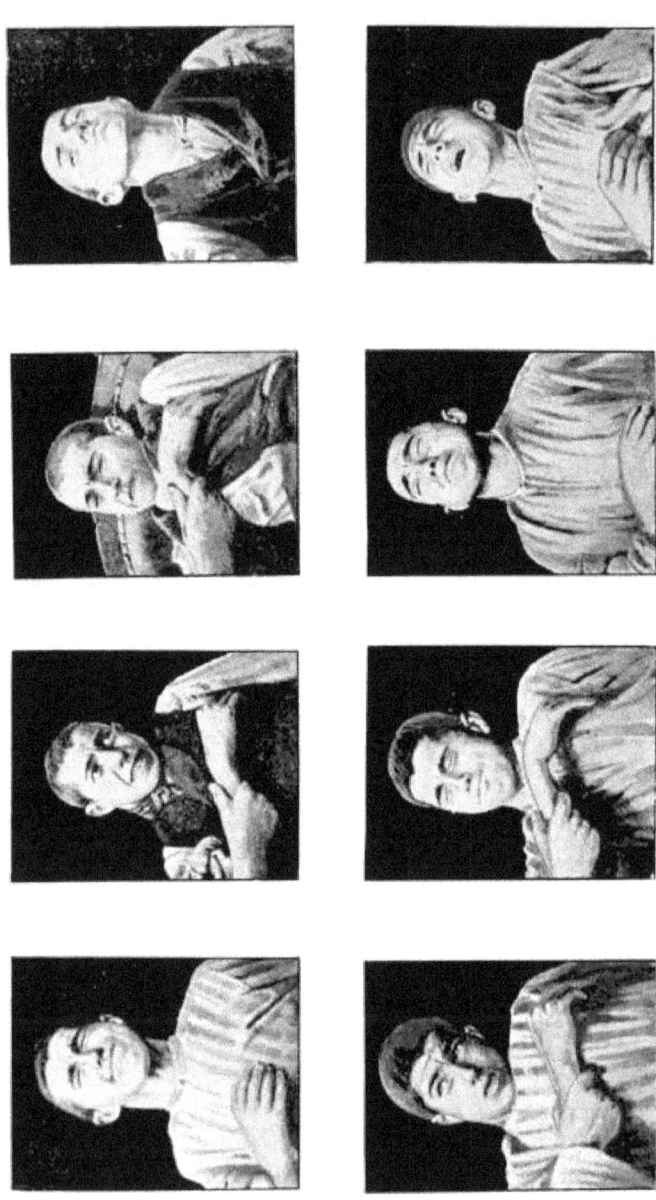

PLATE I.
THE PHYSIOGNOMY OF PAIN

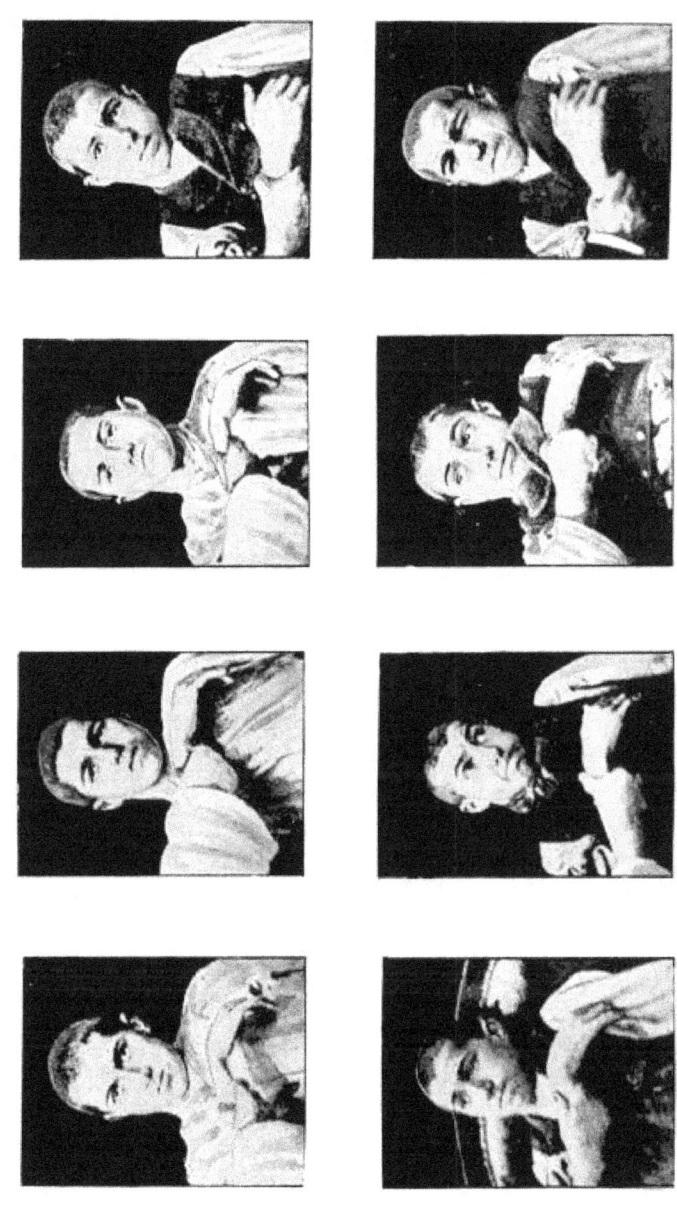

PLATE II.
THE PHYSIOGNOMY OF PAIN

But the contractions of these muscles are no longer of any actual use. When the nerve-force in emotion spreads from the centre towards the periphery, these muscles, from their position in the skin, produce effects which are more easily seen than in other parts of the body, but which serve no effectual purpose in the struggle for existence and in the preservation of life. In the dog and cat, for instance, the contraction of these muscles in strong emotions causes the erection of the hair on the back, and gives the animal the characteristic expression of attack or defence, of fear or pain. In man, on the other hand, a forcible contraction of the cutaneous muscles of the neck which extend under the skin near the lips gives to the mouth the expression so characteristic of children when about to cry, or when they are trying to restrain their tears. Duchenne de Boulogne studied the function of this muscle, and showed that, when irritated by electric currents, it opens the mouth in the manner of one under the influence of terror.

From Ehlers' observations on the facial muscles of the gorilla and chimpanzee, we learn that these animals have the same muscles of the face as we have. Ehlers maintains that the statement made by certain authors is not true, namely, that the single fasciculi in the muscular system of the face of these animals are less thick and compact than in man. Only the wrinklings of the brow are less developed, and the muscles round the eye are finer, while those distributed to the nostrils and lips are more highly developed.

It is not true that laughing and weeping are exclusively human. One need only observe attentively the face of a sensitive and faithful dog in order to see the first traces of expressions betraying an altered state of the nervous system. In joyful emotion, as, for instance, when he meets his master, the lips are lifted in such a manner as to uncover the teeth, the head inclines in a caressing attitude, the rhythm of the respiration is modified, and the eyes glisten. Notwithstanding the difference of anatomical structure and the wide dissimilarity of parts, we can yet trace in the dog the rudiments of those involuntary muscular movements which attain their supreme expression in man, in whom a slight movement of the muscles curves the lips into a smile which sheds a ray of benevolence over the whole face and increases the charm of beauty, as though with the breath of love itself.

Darwin wrote many interesting pages about the way in which monkeys laugh. Humboldt observed the eyes of a monkey fill with tears when it was overcome by fear, and Brehm relates that seals weep with pain, and that young elephants when ill-treated shed tears as abundantly as man.

V

Their reasons why changes in the psychical state are reflected are numerous with such facility by the muscles of the face. Besides that of proximity to the nerve-centres propounded by Spencer and Darwin, there is the anatomical fact that the facial muscles have, for the most part, no antagonists. We know that in the hand, for instance, a slight contraction of the muscles which serve to open the hand and extend the fingers, is opposed by the action of the flexors which bend and contract the fingers. In the face the majority of the muscles can act freely, hence a slight nervous shock produces effects far more intense than in the other muscles of the body, in which the slight contraction of muscles acting in a contrary sense must always be overcome.

The muscles of the face are also more delicate, and have less volume than those of other parts of the body. Now the volume of the muscles exercises considerable influence on the greater or lesser facility with which they contract. A convincing proof is offered by the heart, in which, when life ceases, there is an almost immediate stoppage of the action of the ventricles, which form a thick, firm muscle, while the auricles, forming a fine muscle, continue to move for hours after all other parts are rigid in death.

Another anatomical fact of the greatest importance, brought into prominence by Meynart, is to be found in the origin of the facial nerve within the brain. All other nerves have a very intricate course, and are connected with other cells, and other nerve-filaments, which constitute the cerebral convolutions; the facial nerve only receives commands directly from the central parts of the brain and transmits them by the shortest route to the periphery. If I may allow myself to make use of a comparison, I should say that the facial nerve is like a telegraph wire, which transmits the messages directly to their destination, while with the other nerves the messages are sent successively from one station to another, consequently they pass less rapidly from the brain to their destination in the muscles.

The investigation of that part of the brain whence are issued the commands causing the contraction of the muscles, the accurate, microscopic examination of the cells which, by their activity in the deep parts of the brain, produce the expression of the physiognomy, is a new and important study.

An American anatomist, Mr. Edward Spitzka,[25] discovered that the facial nerve originates in two masses of nerve-cells, called, in anatomical language, nuclei.

There is a lower nucleus, the cells of which preside over the respiratory movements and the expression of the emotions, and an upper nucleus directing the orbicular muscle of the eye. While the latter presents very few variations when studied in different animals of the zoological series, the lower nucleus of the facial nerve, on the other hand, varies considerably, according to the development of the other muscles of the face.

In reptiles, for instance, the nucleus of the facial nerve which goes to the eye is well developed, while the lower nucleus is in a retrograde condition. In birds, which, like reptiles, have no muscles giving expression to the face, this mass of cells forming the lower nucleus is entirely lacking. In the elephant, on the other hand, the lower

[25] Edward C. Spitzka: *Journal of Nervous and Mental Disease*, 1879, s. 69.

nucleus is well developed, because the nose is a complex organ requiring a special group of nerve-cells and nerves in order to act.

Spitzka's anatomical researches having shown that the lower nucleus of the facial nerve reaches its maximum development in the monkey and in man, we must regard it as very probable that the nerve-cells which we see at this point in the brain, at the lower origin of the facial nerve, are really those which produce the expression of the physiognomy.

As I write this, I have before me a very thin section of the brain, showing the nucleus of the facial nerve as it appears in man. It is a gray spot, as large as the head of a small pin, slightly spindle-shaped, and having a volume of about two cubic millimetres. If we look at it under the microscope we see nothing but an accumulation of cells, about the five-hundredths of a millimetre in diameter, and with delicate branches intertwining with each other. In vain the eye tries to find a path through this intricate network of filaments and cells; imagination loses itself as in a labyrinth, and we remain humbled and almost frightened at the thought that we are contemplating the corpse of the noblest part of the brain. The activity of these cells has roused the most powerful emotions of our life: our knowledge of men, our sympathy, indifference, suspicion were provoked by the movements which they gave to the faces of those we have known; friendship, affection, and the most holy joys of life brightened our countenance with a smile which came from these cells; they, again, diffused the shadow of sadness, pain, and tears—and all this drew life from a part of the brain so minute that by a mere touch we could unconsciously crush it.

VI

The greatest difficulties in the study of the alterations which the human face undergoes in suffering are essentially two in number. The first is the rapidity and the perpetual restlessness of muscular movements, which are so fugitive that our eye cannot grasp and comprehend them. The second difficulty lies in the nature of our mind, which is disturbed and touched at the sight of pain. Even men who have been hardened and accustomed to the sight of blood and of human misfortunes, are yet moved at the terrible picture of pain wreaking its rude will on a sensitive organism. Human pain is of such importance that all scientific curiosity becomes a trifling and ridiculous thing, and our mind rebels and feels an invincible repugnance to every desire which has not the alleviation of the sufferer for its object, to every act which does not spring from a lively and intense compassion.

For this reason I made use of instantaneous photographs in studying the expression of the face. The first experiments were made on a few friends and on myself. Pain was produced by introducing the fingers between five pieces of wood, which were then pressed firmly together. This pressure may become unbearable, but the expression of the face is less characteristic than we are accustomed to see in suffering people. In oppression and fear there is not generally that effort of will which subdues the reflex movements in voluntary pain. Tears, agitation, spasms, terror, faintness, which appear in the terrible reality of nature, can only be studied in actual sufferers. I had therefore to leave my laboratory and continue my investigations in the hospitals. I owe thanks to my colleagues in Turin who assisted me during these researches, and allowed me to place my camera in such a position that I could photograph their patients during surgical operations without their being aware of it. The machine opened and closed instantaneously by means of an electric apparatus which I had constructed for this purpose. I could stand near the patient during the operation, and at a given moment, by touching a button, I obtained a picture of the invalid in the camera, which was at a distance of a few paces.

In this way I have made an album of pain. It is a saddening and terrible book, from which I take only two pages, reproduced in Plates I. and II. Their reality is represented in it with such vividness that one shudders on opening it. No artist's fancy has ever been able to imagine or express what photography faithfully reproduces. In acute stages of suffering the human face inspires fear in one contemplating it; it is not alone the profound commiseration which we feel for the anguish of a sentient being which moves us, nor the humiliation which the sight of human misery awakes in us, but also the selfish thought that this palpitating flesh might be our flesh, that our soul, shaken with pain, would also forget its tranquillity, and our tortured nerves wring from us the same cries and the same tears.

The pictures which I reproduce were taken in the Mauriziano hospital in Turin, and represent a boy, eighteen years of age, who had received a wound on his elbow which had healed badly, rendering the joint stiff and leaving the arm bent at a right angle. When he came to Turin, the treatment was begun at once, the arm being moved and stretched daily in order to overcome the resistance and render the joint movable. I photographed the boy twice nearly every day for several weeks, whenever the surgeon forcibly extended the arm, which was intensely painful.

I shall not attempt to describe these pictures, because I feel sure that no words of mine could express the transformation which the human face undergoes in pain. Even had I the talent and the pen of a great artist or a great writer, I should yet refrain, for I know that every description is useless, pale, and vague when confronted with reality. Instantaneous photographs are the best means of showing how even the greatest painters and sculptors have fallen far short of reality, in their representations of the spasms and sufferings which disfigure and distort the human face.

VII

The expression of pain alters according to age; it is different in the child, the youth, the adult, and the old. Energy of will or weakness of character also exercise a profound influence upon it.

I have been present at surgical operations, and have performed them, on persons who refused to be chloroformed, and have noticed how great was the difference of conduct. An old officer, who bore the operation of lithotomy without anæsthetics, only clenched his hands and his teeth, keeping his eyes closed and his face almost impassive. A labourer, whose foot had to be amputated, frowned during the operation, and tapped lightly with curved fingers on the coverlet. There are patients who gnash their teeth, others who roll their eyes upwards, others again who puff; some say, before the operation begins, that they would lie still if only they were allowed to scream.

But none, whatever be the strength of will, succeed in suppressing completely the expression of pain when intense. Only very energetic persons succeed in preserving immovable the muscles of the face, while they discharge the activity of the nervous system into other muscles by tetanic contractions.

We may say that every malady has its peculiar expression of pain. Often, by merely looking at the patient and hearing him moan, the physician can tell which are the affected organs.

This study is very much complicated because of the rare occurrence of simple sensations of pain. Our states of mind are so variable and so complex, that the expression of the face is, as it were, the result of numerous factors. To be convinced we need only think of the touching sight of a woman about to become a mother. Notwithstanding the pangs that torture her, in spite of the indescribable agony of the most intense pains to which human nature is condemned, she yet finds a smile which expresses the hope of surviving, and the joy of motherhood shines in the tender radiance of her eyes, beautifying the face furrowed by cruel suffering.

Italian literature can boast of two very valuable books on the physiology of pain. The first was written by Professor Filippo Lussana in 1860, and dedicated to Dr. Paolo Mantegazza, 'who was writing his celebrated "Physiology of Pleasure" when the joyous spring of his twenty-second year smiled upon the author.' Twenty years later, in 1880, Paolo Mantegazza also published a valuable book on the 'Physiology of Pain.' The merits of this book are great, and it is perhaps one of his greatest achievements in the field of physiology, but science has since made such rapid progress, that it would be well if a third volume were added to the group, developing the anatomical and physiological part, illustrating by instantaneous photographs the most characteristic movements and expressions of pain, and subjecting to a severe criticism the most celebrated pictures and statues of the various schools. I cherish the wish that Paolo Mantegazza, who was my master, and one of the greatest popularisers of science, may find time to complete and rejuvenate his work, for who else would find courage to take a place at his side, and to glean where he has reaped?

VIII

The art of the future, comprising all visible nature within its limits, will find a great and terrible potency of effect in the expression of pain. The difficulties, certainly, are here much greater than in the calm reproduction of the ideally beautiful, and those painters and sculptors who wish to grapple with the problem of the expression of pain must train themselves by the study of reality, and arm themselves with anatomical and physiological knowledge of which antique art gives us no example.

I believe that, with the advance of a scientific criticism nurtured on an accurate knowledge of physiology, and intimately acquainted with the functions of the muscles, we shall one day recognise that the Greeks of the epoch of Phidias and Praxiteles were unequal to the effectual reproduction of violent passions.

Winckelmann said that Greek art was always tranquil and majestic, like the depths of the sea, which remain immovably calm, however the tempest may ruffle the surface. But I fear there is some exaggeration in the statement that beauty was the only law of Greek art, and that the Greeks shunned the expression of pain because the sight of suffering excites disgust in the spectator. Sophocles and Homer believed in an art of wider limits; they made their heroes weep, and shriek, and groan; all human weaknesses are faithfully represented by them, descending even to the grotesque and ridiculous. At the epoch of Phidias monuments vividly expressing the internal passions of the soul are rare. It was only later, in the time of Praxiteles and Scopas, that subjects and compositions of greater effect were attempted. The most ancient monument of pain, that representing the destruction of Niobe's children, does not attain the perfection of other famous works of that epoch. The subject is tragic in the highest degree, and such that one cannot say the Greeks shunned the terrific. It may be that the statue of the Niobe in Florence is a bad copy, but it is much more probable that the artists of that epoch, who were unrivalled and beyond all rivalry in the representation of grace of attitude and silent majesty, could not touch with the same master-hand the other chords to which the human heart vibrates.

Some great artist—perhaps Praxiteles or Scopas—wished to adorn the temple of Apollo with this terrible picture of revenge taken upon man by an offended deity. It is Niobe, the daughter of Tantalus, who, proud of her children, dared to compare herself to the mother of Apollo, and now sees them killed one after another, shot by the revengeful arrows of Apollo and Artemis. No subject could be more tragic. The first time I entered the 'Galleria degli Uffizi' in Florence, I remember halting, almost afraid, at the door leading to the hall of the Niobean group, thinking of the heart-rending scene I was about to see, and of the emotion which I should feel while contemplating one of the most celebrated productions of Greek art. I confess that it did not produce the effect which I had imagined, and that a careful examination of the statues forming the group resulted in a great disappointment.

Only the mother filled me with emotion, so perfect is her attitude, so real her gesture; but in her face and in that of her children there is no true reflection of the awful event taking place. There is no physiological correspondence in the pose of the limbs and between the muscles of the body and those of the face. There is insufficient accuracy in the sculpture of the heads, for in them is lacking the expression of intense emotion, of horror, fear, and pain which would inevitably be present in the terrible moment of so cruel a butchery. Even though the convulsions and spasms had altered the beauty of the lines to which the eye of the Greeks was accustomed, it was yet the duty of the artist faithfully to represent reality. Nor can it be said that the artist feared to fall into the grotesque, because certain postures of the children are so violent, that in their boldness they perhaps exaggerate the truth. Though Praxiteles himself were the creator of the Niobean group, I yet hold that a humble physiologist, looking with dispassionate eye at these statues, may affirm that they fall short of the fame of so great a master, because the faces are not so modelled as to produce the desired effect, because nature is not faithfully copied, and because there lacks the sublime ideality of terror aroused by the chastisement of an offended deity, which was the subject of the work.

It was in the schools of Asia Minor, after the time of Alexander, in Pergamos and Rhodes, that antique art, before it became extinct, developed its greatest splendour, showing an irresistible tendency to the representation of pain. It is to the school of Rhodes that the Laocoon group belongs. So much has been written about this celebrated work, that I should have nothing to add if the face of Laocoon were anatomically correct. Duchenne de Boulogne was the first to notice the defects of the Laocoon of Rome, and to declare that the furrows of the brow in this celebrated statue are physiologically impossible. The eye of the superficial observer does not notice this defect, because the movement of the eyebrows which produces the fundamental line of pain is marvellously modelled. Some perhaps will say that it is useless to stop to criticise the delineation of a few furrows when such an intense and majestic pain is written on the face, when one seems to hear the sigh of superhuman agony from his lips, and sees the lines of beauty and of pain so wonderfully blended.

The discoveries which have been made of late years in the excavations in the Acropolis of Pergamos have restored to the admiration of centuries treasures which mark an epoch in the history of plastic art, and throw a vivid light on the last phase with which Greek art completed its evolution. Works so moving as those of the sculptors of Pergamos had never been produced before. Art devoted itself entirely to the embodiment and representation of physical pain in its innumerable manifestations, as though the observation and experience of suffering, the study of the pathetic, having accumulated for centuries in the mind of artists and people, burst forth impetuously at the sight of the victories over the barbarians who threatened their country with invasion. We have in Italy some of the most celebrated masterpieces of the school of Pergamos. As all know them I shall only mention the statue of the dying Gaul in the Museo Capitolino. The head is not so beautiful as those of the Greek statues, but, on the other hand, it wears so vivid an expression of pain that we feel touched at the brave death of this barbarian, who breathes his last leaning upon his shield, while the blood gushes from the fatal wound. This statue, together with the group in the Villa Ludovisi to which it belongs, was placed on the Acropolis of Pergamos about 200 years before the vulgar era, in order to celebrate the victory of Attalus I. over the barbarians. In the second group we have again a barbarian before

112

us, who, pursued by an enemy, kills his wife, and then with the same dagger, as he looks behind him, his eyes wild with the fear that the enemy may be near and make him a prisoner before he dies, he stabs himself.

Brizio, in his 'Studies of the Laocoon,' speaking of the school of Pergamos, says: 'After an exhaustive examination of the statues in the museums of Naples, Venice, Rome, and St. Germain-en-Laye, not only the intention of the artists becomes evident, but also the pleasure they took in representing with the greatest perspicuity the death of combatants with all the torture and agony preceding it. In none of the monuments prior to this epoch is anything similar to be found, although Greek sculpture, beginning with Phidias, boasts a conspicuous series of representations of combats. In all these scenes the artists endeavoured to find new situations, to recreate and vary the groups of combatants, to reproduce the ardour of the fight; they even represented the wounded and the dead, but simply as episodes; they never made a study of death itself, of its tragic effects, with the manifest object of moving and exciting to the highest degree the compassion of the spectator. In these groups death is rather indicated than represented.

A further step in the representation of physical pain is marked by the sculpture of the 'War of the Titans' around the altar of Jove. When we throw a comprehensive glance on these scenes of the battle between gods and giants, we are struck by a new and horrible phenomenon—namely, the part which the animals, tearing the human bodies to pieces, take in it.

Anyone contemplating in the Museum of Berlin the figures in haut-relief which formerly adorned the plinth of the altar at Pergamos, 135 metres in length, feels that this is perhaps the most imposing work which sculpture has ever produced. Art was in full possession of its most potent means, and more advanced science had contributed its part. It was by a most minute study of details, by an exact knowledge of the movements of the muscles, and long practice in the observation of the physiognomy of passion, that antique plastic art, in the last period of its splendour, attained its highest effect in the expression of feeling. This, I think, is the natural law in the evolution of art.

CHAPTER XII

A FEW PHENOMENA CHARACTERISTIC OF FEAR

I

The edifice of the human body may be compared by those studying its chemical processes to a vast manufactory of which every corner and every door bears the inscription, 'NO ADMITTANCE.' The curiosity of the public could not be greater; fain would they force an entrance, for all know that the most marvellous things are fabricated therein—wonders which no human hand, no industry, can produce.

The workmen in this factory are very small—marvellously small—invisible to the naked eye, and so tightly pressed together that they sometimes resemble the cells of a beehive, and have, on this account, received the name of cells. Life proceeds entirely from these workmen, whose confederation is so perfect that not one can be touched without the others at once becoming aware of it.

The edifice is somewhat weak in parts, and here one might easily force an entrance and make a wide breach; but this violence would avail us little, for when we break into the building the machines stop, causing such disorder and confusion that we are quite bewildered. We hear a whirring and throbbing, the pipes burst, the fluids are spilt, the pumps stop, the valves open—then all grows cold and still; and this is the strike which we call death.

The history of the attempts made to discover the actual nature of the activity of these workmen who keep the secret of life is one of the most beautiful studies in science; in reading it, there comes over us a feeling of admiration and gratitude towards those men who, in all ages, have spent their whole life in investigations, accumulating experience, sacrificing worldly goods and honours for one little gleam of light, defying poverty and toil, making the hardest and most cruel sacrifices for the sake of one forward step, of lifting but a little the mysterious veil, sometimes only to stretch out a hand to help others to walk over their body.

Thousands of volumes have been written about this struggle, and those who only read an epitome of it in the treatises of physiological chemistry are yet astonished at the power of the human mind, and at the incredible, almost superhuman, difficulties with which it has to cope.

Never was there, nor will there be, any war even faintly resembling in ardour, perseverance, and power of intellectual means, this siege of centuries, which seeks to close every issue to Nature and force her to reveal the secret of her chemical operations.

It is wonderful to see how attacks are prepared in advance, what cunning traps are laid, and by what subtle signs the road of ingress is divined. Who can describe the joy of all besiegers when one step forward has been made, or a glimmer of light is detected in the darkness? The exultation and applause which welcome every invention which resolves, or analyses, or recomposes a molecule, every instrument which enables us to break one crumb off the immense rock of the Unknown? And who shall tell the tale of pain, of disappointment, bitterness, and error; of the forgotten or unknown deeds of heroism, of existences lost in the obscurity of the schools, of the laboratories, of the hospitals; of those who die unnoticed in these last trenches where spectators and witnesses to shout applause are lacking?

And yet this deters no one; all press onward. The soldiers of science renew their vigilance and redouble their caution, the phalanx of the living draws closer together, returning with fresh courage to the assault.

Nothing can resist this unremitting war, this wonderful harmony of aim, this iron will of man; we will die on the battle-field with the certainty that others will take up our weapons and that the victory will be ours.

II

The prohibition to enter the manufactory of the human body is not so strict but that we may advance a little. We can see everything which goes in, that is, certain substances called food, which we all know, because they are publicly offered for sale; nor is it difficult to obtain permission to follow them through the mouth which forms the entry, and a long corridor, called the œsophagus, into a large, damp, warm cavity called the stomach, in which all substances are reduced to a very fine pulp; the whitish juice runs into certain little canals which flow into the circulating stream called blood, of which we have already spoken, and out of which every workman, every cell, draws what is necessary for its work. But no one has ever really discovered what is done with this appropriated material—the manner of its digestion and elaboration.

We know that the motor force of the manufactory is due to a change—a chemical operation, by which the energy of the substances introduced is transformed and appropriated by the cells that manifest it externally in that force which we call muscular contraction cerebral activity, &c.

The most important chemical operations performed in the manufactory are three in number. The first consists in the transformation of food into protoplasm, or cell-substance; the second, in the discharge of the energy accumulated in these cells; the third, in the elimination of those substances which the cells have exhausted and rendered useless.

If we make a careful comparison, by means of chemical analysis, between the composition of the substances introduced and those eliminated, we always find that the chemical energy of the latter is much reduced, from which we may know that it is food which puts everything in movement, for with nothing, nothing is made.

The walls of the building are often moistened by a fluid which trickles through in drops, and is called perspiration. Physiologists have constructed most costly apparatus in order to collect the smoke of the chimney and the air which escapes from the mouths of the innumerable ventilators called pores. Every little thing was studied and conscientiously analysed, and all were surprised that these elaborate and most intricate operations of life should result finally in products so simple. We may say that our body only produces carbonic acid, urea, and a few salts.

III

Let us enter more fully into this subject, so that we may understand the meaning of certain phenomena accompanying fear.

The materials rendered useless in the operations of our factory are easily eliminated through the skin, which thus co-operates in one of the most important functions, that of internal cleansing, which is more particularly the office of the kidneys.

We have all observed that we usually perspire when the skin is red; but there are exceptional cases, as in fear, when we perspire, although we are pale and trembling. How does it happen that we have a cold perspiration, and a perspiration with a sensation of warmth in the skin? I shall here mention an experiment of Claude Bernard. Having severed a filament of the sympathetic nerves on the neck of a horse, he saw immediately afterwards, although the animal had not moved, an abundant secretion on that half of its head where the cut had been made. The mechanism producing this phenomenon is easily understood: as soon as the nerve is severed which held the blood-vessels in check, the latter dilate, blood flows more copiously to the sudoriparous glands, increasing their activity and causing an elimination of the secreted liquid.

When it is warm, or when we are feverish, and the blood tends to flow more abundantly to the surface of the body to cool itself, the secretion of perspiration is increased in a similar way. But we see anæmic persons perspire—the consumptive, for instance, and the dying, in whom this more copious supply of blood is wanting. In this case the cause of abundant secretion is different; here it is the nerves. One of the finest discoveries which have been made of late years in physiology, is that of the nerve-filaments which connect the cerebro-spinal system with the glands of the body. Whereas formerly everything was attributed to the more or less copious flow of blood to the glands, the secretions of which were considered as a process of filtration, we now know that the matter is much more complicated, and that there are nerves which augment and diminish the activity of the cells charged with the secretion. It is nervous activity which produces the perspiration characteristic of attention, pain, epilepsy, tetanus.

In order to prove that the secretion of perspiration may be accomplished independently of the circulation of the blood, we make an incision in the leg of a cat immediately after death and irritate the sciatic nerve; we then see that a secretion of perspiration still appears on the sole of the foot. From this we can understand how in the death-agony and the extreme pallor of fright, when all the vessels of the skin are contracted, there yet may appear a peculiar secretion of perspiration which we call *cold perspiration.*

IV

There is another part of the body which opens periodically to allow of the ejection of the refuse of the factory; it consists in a *cloaca* and a cistern which contains a yellow liquid. It is a less beautiful part of the organism, but during violent emotions involuntary movements are produced in it so characteristic of fear that we must turn our attention to it. Physicians thought that these irregularities were caused by a paralysis of the sphincter muscle, but this is not the case. The researches which I made with Prof. Pellicani[26] showed that, in man as well as in animals, there are strong contractions of the bladder which correspond to psychic facts. Scarcely have we experienced some slight emotion or been excited by some thought but there is an immediate change in the state of the muscles of this organ. I regret that the nature of this book does not permit of the reproduction of the curves traced by the plethysmograph, which show that psychic phenomena and any irritation of the sensory nerves produce a contraction of the bladder.

This is the reason why, during emotion, we feel the urgent and repeated need to expel the urine, without the amount of accumulated liquid being such as to explain the necessity. We can no doubt all remember the annoyance which the contraction of this organ caused us on certain solemn occasions; for instance, when we had to make a speech, or present ourselves for an examination, or were anxiously expecting something.

The feeling of contraction and pressure in the abdomen when we approach a precipice, or when we are in great apprehension, is solely due to the involuntary contraction of the bladder. We have shown that all causes producing a contraction of the blood-vessels have the same effect on the muscles of the bladder. I have often seen excitable, good-tempered dogs, in whom caresses and the sight of food were sufficient to produce such a contraction of the bladder, that the urine was expelled; and this suffices to confirm the fact that in our organism the same phenomena may be produced by opposite causes.

In emotions violently agitating the nervous system, and especially in fear, the contraction of the bladder is so forcible that the will can no longer hinder the expulsion of the accumulated liquid; it is therefore not a paralysis, but too forcible a contraction of the walls of the bladder which causes the involuntary expulsion.

---

[26] Mosso e Pellicani: *Sulle funzioni della vescica.* R. Accademia dei Lincei, vol. xii. 1881.

Let us throw a passing glance at what takes place in the *cloaca maxima*. The intestinal walls are as contractile as those of the bladder; nor need this surprise us, as they are furnished with smooth muscles, and receive nerves and blood-vessels from the same source. We know, indeed, that this canal is subject to rapid movements, for we have all frequently heard that rumbling noise of the intestines which we cannot suppress. If the abdominal walls were transparent, we should see, when this occurs, that there is a limited contraction of the intestinal walls which propagates itself slowly in the direction of the egress. These movements, called peristaltic, are present even when we hear no noise; they serve to mix the food in the stomach, promote digestion, and convey the useless residuum to the rectum.

In paroxysms of fear the rapidity of these movements is so greatly increased that, in a very short time, they convey substances introduced into the stomach to the terminal portion of the intestines before there has been time to elaborate, digest, and condense them. It is therefore no paralysis which may, in certain circumstances, make the most courageous men appear ridiculous, it is a stream overflowing its banks—the intestines contracting so violently as to eject their contents rapidly from the organism.

One of my friends, who served as a volunteer in 1866, described to me the physical disturbances which he suffered the first time he was under fire. 'Believe me,' he said, 'nothing can give you an idea of the furious shower of bullets which whizzed about our ears. We were near a cemetery; perhaps it was the sight of the crosses and of some corpses lying by the road-side which increased my terror, but the bullets burying themselves in the walls and trees, the cries of wounded comrades, the grim rattle of musketry, the roar of the cannon, seemed to tear me inwardly. The dysentery was so terrible that my body seemed to fall to pieces. I was always cowering in the ditches, could only stumble forwards, scarcely even rise from the ground. I was ashamed; I could have killed myself only to be able to look death bravely in the face, but, indeed, my organism could not bear that terrible sight!'

V

A still more characteristic phenomenon in the picture of fear is *goose-skin*. Let us see how and why the skin corrugates in this way. We know that besides the sudoriparous glands there are other glands at the surface of the body which secrete a peculiar fat called *sebum*, which oils the surface of the skin and gives it that gloss which we notice on the face of some people.

If we take a vertical section of the skin, we can see with the microscope a close network of muscular fibres which traverse the skin in an oblique direction, and surround every hair in the manner of the ribs of an umbrella. It is wonderful to see this mechanism under the microscope, how every hair has its own gland, its own muscle and its own nerve, its own arteries and veins. When these muscles contract, the meshes of the skin contract likewise and express the contents of the glands. We do not notice these movements of the skin, because the muscles contract very slowly.

Sometimes special muscles appear in the skin called cutaneous muscles, which play an important part in the life of animals.

We all know how the hedgehog rolls himself into a ball on the approach of danger. This movement, as we have already stated, is executed by means of a muscle covering the whole of the body, like a hood or purse which may be drawn together on one side. In the mole, too, these muscles are very strong, and we have already mentioned that dogs and horses twitch the skin to rid themselves of flies, and that this movement is due to a rapid contraction of one of these muscles. When animals curl themselves up, with the muzzle close to the tail, as the sleeping dog does, head and limbs are more easily held in this position by means of these muscles. I have found them more or less in all superior animals, and shall now consider the possible uses of these muscles which exist also in man.

It does not seem to me correct to say that they serve to drive the flies away, because they are well developed in reptiles and fish, and in many animals of which the skin is insensible to the stings of insects; also, if the fly-hypothesis were the correct one, the cutaneous muscles should be best developed on those parts of the animal which cannot easily be reached with the head, the leg, or the tail, but the contrary is the case.

Certainly the muscles are made use of for this purpose, but this is an accidental fact, as is also, I believe, the circumstance that these muscles serve to erect the hair when the animal is excited or afraid. When one dog approaches another in a hostile mood, there is such an agitation of his nervous system that he begins to tremble, not through fear, but excessive excitement. All the muscles contract, those of the blood-vessels, of the bladder, of the intestines, therefore it is comprehensible that the cutaneous muscles should also contract, raising the hair on the dog's back.

If we look at the skin of the arms or legs when we step into a cold bath, or when we uncover ourselves on rising in the morning while the temperature of the room is low, we notice the appearance of goose-skin.

Whenever there is, for some reason, a contraction of the blood-vessels, these muscles contract also and the hair rises. The simultaneous appearance of these two phenomena is, I believe, useful to the animal, because, in raising the hair or feathers, the stratum of air enclosed by these appendages is increased, the loss of heat in this way diminished, and the cooling of the skin prevented. It is, perhaps, for this reason that horses, dogs, cats, and birds ruffle their hair or feathers when cold.[27]

---

[27] Darwin gives another explanation of this phenomenon which seems to me less probable. He states that animals erect their dermal appendages that they may appear larger and more terrible to their enemies.
But how can it be explained that these smooth muscles should be originally dependent on the will? In order to avoid the doubly improbable supposition that these muscles should have become smooth and involuntary,

although preserving the same functions, Darwin has recourse to another explanation. 'We may admit,' he says, 'that originally the arrectores pili were slightly acted on in a direct manner, under the influence of rage and terror, by the disturbance of the nervous system.' 'Animals have been repeatedly excited by rage and terror through many generations; and consequently the direct effects of the disturbed nervous system on the dermal appendages will almost certainly have been increased through habit and through the tendency of nerve-force to pass readily along accustomed channels.' 'As soon as with animals the power of erection has thus been strengthened or increased, they must often have seen the hairs or feathers erected in rival and enraged males, and the bulk of their bodies thus increased. In this case it appears possible that they might have wished to make themselves appear larger and more terrible to their enemies ... such attitudes and utterances after a time becoming through habit instinctive.'

'It is even possible ... that the will is able to influence in an obscure manner the action of some unstriped or involuntary muscles, as in the period of the peristaltic movements of the intestines, and in the contraction of the bladder.'*

* Ch. Darwin: *The Expression of the Emotions*, p. 103.

CHAPTER XIII

FEAR IN CHILDREN. DREAMS

I

The one who brings up a child represents its brain. Every ugly thing told to the child, every shock, every fright given him, will remain like minute splinters in the flesh, to torture him all his life long.

An old soldier, whom I asked what his greatest fears had been, answered me thus: 'I have only had one, but it pursues me still. I am nearly seventy years old, I have looked death in the face I do not know how many times, I have never lost heart in any danger, but when I pass a little old church in the shades of the forest, or a deserted chapel in the mountains, I always remember a neglected oratory in my native village, and I shiver and look around, as though seeking the corpse of a murdered man which I once saw carried into it when a child, and with which an old servant wanted to shut me up to make me good.'

Anxiety, fear, horror will twine themselves perpetually around the memory, like deadly ivy choking the light of reason. At every step we remember the terrors of childhood: the vaults of a cellar, the dark arch of a bridge, the cross-roads losing themselves in the darkness, the crosses hidden amidst the bushes of a cemetery, a dim light flickering far away in the darkness of night, a lonely cave washed by the waves of the sea, the ruins of an uninhabited castle, the mysterious silence of a deserted tower, breathe out the memory of childish fear. The eye of the child seems to cast one more look on these scenes from out of the very depths of the soul.

Not only the mother, the nurse, the maid, or the servants, but hundreds of generations have worked to denaturalise the brains of children with the same barbarity as those wild tribes who distort the heads of their children by pressure, deforming what they think to beautify.

The children of ancient Greece and Rome used to be frightened with the lamias who would suck their blood, with the masks of the atellans, the Cyclops, or with a black Mercury who would come to carry them away.

And this most pernicious error in education has not yet disappeared, for children are still frightened with the bogey-man, with stories of imaginary monsters, the ogre, the hobgoblin, the wizard, and the witches.

Every now and then children are told: 'This will peck at you,' 'That will bite you,' 'Now I'll call the dog,' 'There's the sweep coming,' and a hundred other terrors which make the tears well up and spoil their disposition, making their life a burden by incessantly agitating them with threats, with tortures, which will make them timid and shrinking for the rest of their life.

The imagination of children is far more vivid and excitable than in adults. When a child is naturally timorous, it is better not to leave it in the dark, but to keep a night-light burning in the room, so that, on waking, it may at once recognise the place, and its fancies may not assume an air of reality. The child's eye is much more apt than ours to trace pursuing spectres in the outlines of accustomed objects. The stories told them in the evening, any exciting emotions towards night-time, are most certainly reproduced in their dreams.

A turkey-cock, ten days old, that had never heard the cry of the falcon, disappeared with the rapidity of lightning when it heard the cry the first time, hiding itself in a corner, where it cowered motionless and silent for more than ten minutes.

Spalding took a brood of chickens, a week old, and while they were chirping around the hen in the meadow, he let fly a falcon. At once the chickens tried to hide in the grass and bushes, and the hen, that had always been kept shut up, so that she might have no experience of enemies, precipitated herself with such violence on the falcon on seeing it that she would certainly have killed it. Now neither she nor her first brood had ever seen a bird of prey. Spalding, in order to assure himself that it really is instinct which causes the recognition of enemies, had already let some pigeons fly, and these settled near the hen without producing any disturbance or emotion, as in the case of the falcon. We must therefore admit that there is an innate recollection which constitutes fear.

II

Philosophers, always dominated by a sublime idea of human faculties, have too much neglected the study of savages and children. And yet it is here that we ought to begin, if it is true that one must proceed from the simple to the complex. Physiologists seem, more than others, to have recognised this necessity, in order to distinguish inherited psychic facts from those which we are capable of acquiring by the experience of the senses. Let the physiologist remain long days at home with a sympathetic wife and a darling child, attentively observing and writing the whole life of the latter; this is for him the best, the ideal study.

My colleague, Prof. Preyer, one of the most distinguished of embryologists, had this happy thought, and his book on the 'Soul of the Child'[28] is one of the most interesting volumes of modern psychology.

Even the first day after birth the face of the child changes suddenly if it is held towards the light from the window, or if its eyes are shaded by a hand.

On the second day it shuts its eyes forcibly and immediately when a lighted candle is brought near to it, and draws its head back energetically if a light is held before its eyes on waking.

---

[28] Preyer: *Die Seele des Kindes.* Jena, 1882.

In this case the child responds through excessive sensitiveness, not through fear. A child, a few months old, looking at the clouds or a snow-covered surface, closes its eyes oftener and more forcibly than an adult.

During the first month children do not wink at a sudden noise, or when one makes a pretence of putting a finger into their eye.

In Prof. Preyer's child this movement appeared for the first time on the fifty-seventh day, and only from the sixtieth did it become regular and constant. We cannot think that a child, nine weeks old, can have any conception of danger, and that it closes its eyes and lifts its hands from fear. It was certainly not the result of experience, as we know that there had been no opportunity for it to learn the injurious nature of many things.

Instead of entertaining the notion of fear, it seems more logical to consider these facts as analogous to the shutting of the eyes during the first hours of life.

The sudden shadow or sound constitutes a disagreeable fact, and the disturbed nervous system responds by a reflex movement, just as many children cry when they hear the first clap of thunder, although they do not know what it is, and start when they suddenly hear a door bang or some object fall.

Preyer noticed that in the seventh week his child started and lifted its hands at any sudden noise without waking.

An expression of the greatest wonder can be produced in a child of seven months old by opening and shutting a fan before it; but the wide-open eye and mouth and the fixed look are not merely signs of astonishment, for when one draws the infant away from the breast, it expresses its lively desire to be fed again by the same attitude.

In these cases the eyes shine with a more abundant secretion of tears. Wide-open eyes accompany the first smile. One notices that children have a tendency to open their eyes in joy and close them in displeasure.

Children, like the insane and like animals, when they have had some disagreeable experience, are frightened at everything which they do not know. Sometimes fear appears suddenly; from one day to another a child may become timid and frightened when it sees an unknown person, or if the father or mother makes some unusual gesture, or calls loudly.

The fear which children have of dogs and cats, before they have learnt why they are to be feared, is a consequence of heredity; even later, when they have gained some experience, they are overcome with fear at the sight of sucking pups or kittens, which would be ridiculous if it were not an innate aversion. The same may be said of the fear of falling when they make the first steps, although they have never yet fallen, and of the fear which children have at the first sight of the sea.

III

Pavor nocturnus is a malady peculiar to children from the third to the seventh year, and must not be confounded with nightmare.

The symptoms are the following: Sudden awaking of the child after a few hours of profound sleep.—A vivid expression of great terror, the eyes fixed on some point, as though on some apparition standing before them.—Failure of consciousness: the child recognises no one, and does not reply to questions.—Skin bathed in perspiration.—Stronger cardiac pulsations.—Rapid pulse.—Laboured breath.—Trembling of the limbs.—Temperature normal.

The intensity, duration, and frequency of these attacks vary greatly; they last generally from five to twenty minutes, after which the children recover consciousness and fall asleep.

In the morning they remember nothing. Rarely do the attacks occur several times in the same night; they appear as a rule at intervals of a few days, often disappearing altogether after occurring two or three times.

The causes of this malady are hereditary or accidental. Pale, delicate, thin, scrofulous, anæmic, very intelligent or irritable children are easily attacked; predisposed to it also are children of excitable parents, or of those troubled with nervous affections. Amongst occasional causes of the *pavor nocturnus* may be specially mentioned strong emotions, fever, and diseases of the digestive organs. In general the children recover; the prognosis, as we say, is favourable.

Some retain their excessive nervous excitability, are subject to palpitation of the heart, but only in very exceptional conditions have the attacks of *pavor nocturnus* exercised a lastingly injurious influence.

IV

The dreams of children are more real, vivid, fearful than of adults, because their brain is excessively impressionable, as is shown by the fact that things seen in childhood are indelibly impressed on the memory, and because their life is made up of emotions, while their weakness renders them more timorous, exaggerates every danger, and makes every enemy appear disproportionately superior to them in strength.

Emotions and fright may become so great in dreams that some children have had actual epileptic fits in consequence, as has recently been proved by Prof. Nothnagel.

In adults dreams seem sometimes so vividly real, that they resemble delirious paroxysms. What terrible events have taken place, what catastrophes at which we shudder, recognising the fragility of the human mind and the awful power of dreams!

I quote a single case which took place in Glasgow in 1878.

A man, twenty-four years old, of the name of Fraser, rose suddenly during the night, took his child and hurled it against the wall, shattering its skull. The screams of his wife awakened him, when, to his horror, he found that he had killed his son whom he had thought to save from a wild animal which he had seen enter the room and spring on to the child's bed to devour it. Fraser gave himself up to justice at once and was set at liberty, because it was evident that he had acted unconsciously.

He was a workman, pale, of a nervous temperament, sluggish intellect, and rather childish, but industrious at his work. His mother had suffered all her life from epileptic attacks, eventually dying in a fit of this kind. His father, too, was epileptic. His maternal aunt and her children were insane; his sister died, as a child, in convulsions. From his infancy he had been the victim of terrifying dreams, in which he used to spring, screaming, out of bed. These dreams troubled him especially when he had suffered any emotion during the day. He had once saved his little sister from falling into the water, and this had made such an impression on him that he often rose during the night, called loudly to his sister, and clasped her in his arms as though to keep her from falling. Sometimes he would awake, sometimes go back to bed, still sleeping, and in the morning would feel depressed without remembering anything. After his marriage in 1875 the attacks assumed a different character.

He was pursued by terrible dreams, and used to spring out of bed screaming 'Fire!' or that his son was in convulsions, or that a wild animal had got into the room, which he would then try to find and hit with anything which fell into his hands. Several times he had seized his wife, his father, and a friend who lived with him, by the throat, nearly strangling them in the belief that he had caught the wild animal. In these attacks his eyes were wide-open and full of expression, and he saw all objects, although he was blind to everything which did not agree with his mental illusions. It was in one of these attacks that he killed his son.

And he was an affectionate father! The mind shudders at the thought of his unspeakable grief when consciousness returned.

CHAPTER XIV

FRIGHT AND TERROR

I

One of the most terrible effects of fear is the paralysis which allows neither of escape nor defence.

The history of battles and massacres, the chronicles of the courts of justice, are full of frightful occurrences when terror strangled even the instinct of flight in the victim.

But how does it happen that under the influence of a powerful emotion the empire of the will over the muscles ceases, and the energy for defence fails?

If we study the phenomena of sleep, we can easily imagine that there are links between the centres of the will and the muscles which may, in certain circumstances, be severed. We all know what nightmare is; we all remember the oppression we have suffered when, in a dream, we have felt ourselves suffocating under an immovable weight on the chest, or from a noose round the throat which we cannot unloose. These dreams, in which we feel ourselves paralysed, are a positive torture; the ground gives way under us and we are precipitated into an abyss; we fall while being pursued and cannot get up again; we find ourselves stretched out in the middle of the street and hear the approaching roll of wheels that will crush us, or see a horse gallop up to trample us with its hoofs. We cannot even scream, hands and feet try in vain to move, the oppression and despair increase until the nightmare passes and we awake with beating heart and laboured breath.

Women and children overcome by violent fear turn their back, cover their eyes with their hands, or creep into a corner without looking behind them. In terror even the most intrepid men do not think of flight; it seems as though the nerves of defence were severed and they were left to their fate. Even in slight emotions we notice a partial failure of the power of the will over the muscles of the hand. Anyone weeping bitterly or laughing heartily cannot steady the pen between the fingers, and the writing is altered.

Whytt noticed that after the head is cut off an animal, its excitability increases greatly after the lapse of a few minutes. The electric stimuli applied to the skin of the trunk immediately after decapitation do not produce any movement of reaction, but a few minutes later the same electric current causes vigorous movements of the legs.

This unexpected phenomena gave rise to the belief that there were mechanisms in the spinal cord which, when irritated by the violent blow of the axe, were capable of arresting the reflex movements. But there are many other experiments which lead us rather to suspect the existence in the nerve-centres of some mechanism which, in certain conditions, nullifies the power of the will over the muscles.

Anyone who has tritons in an aquarium can try the experiment of seizing hold of one by the leg with a pair of pincers; he will see that it remains motionless, almost rigid, for a few minutes. Frogs, when suffering a strong irritation of the sensory nerves, are no longer capable of making a single movement. There are also many other experiments which show us how, under the influence of violent and supernormal excitation, the molecular work of the cells of the spinal cord, requisite for the production of muscular movement through voluntary stimuli, is impeded.

II

Horses tremble when they see a tiger, and are no longer able to run. Even monkeys cannot move when in great fear. The gibbons, the most agile of all monkeys, when taken by surprise on the ground, passively allow themselves to be bound by man. Seals become so agitated when surprised and pursued on shore, that they fall at every step, snort, tremble, and cannot defend themselves.

I quote a passage taken from Brehm's 'Animal Life,' in order to show in what an ignoble way man makes use of the disastrous effects which fright produces. Seals are very intelligent animals, and so good-tempered, that on lonely islands they look with the utmost indifference at travellers arriving there, and such is their trust, that they tranquilly allow them to pass or stop in their midst, while they sun themselves on the shore. But as soon as they learn from sad experience to know this terrible destroyer of animals, they become so cautious that they are with difficulty approached or surprised out of the water.

'To the south of Santa Barbara, in California, there is a plateau, rising about thirty metres above the level of the sea, which is a favourite place of repose with the seals. As soon as the boats were lowered, the animals descended from the plateau and plunged into the sea, where they stayed till all danger was over and the crew reassembled on board. The attempt to surprise them was repeatedly made without success, until one day, when a fresh wind was blowing from the plateau towards the ship, and a thick fog afforded effectual concealment. The crew landed at a certain distance, and, keeping to leeward, crept cautiously up to the herd, then rushed suddenly upon them, shouting noisily and brandishing guns, clubs, and spears. Overwhelmed with fear, with staring eyes, their tongues hanging out of their open mouths, the poor animals remained motionless, petrified, until at last the oldest and most courageous males tried to break through the line of destroyers who closed the way towards the sea. But they were killed before they reached the water, the crew then slowly approaching the others, which retreated just as slowly. An attack of this kind soon becomes a butchery, because the poor animals lose all hope of escape, and abandon themselves helplessly to their fate. This herd numbered seventy-five seals, and when all had been killed with clubs and spears but one single animal, the crew thought to try whether it would allow itself to be driven on without resistance. Forced on by its cruel persecutors, the poor creature moved as well as it could over the thorns and undergrowth, until at last, wounded and bleeding, it stopped, stretched out its fins full of thorns to the sailors, as though to move them to pity and beg for mercy. A blow from a club on its head put an end to its sufferings.'[29]

And this is Man!

III

Fear is more manifest in birds than in any other animal. We sometimes see jugglers, as a proof of their magic power, take a little bird in their hand and lay it on its back, showing that it no longer moves, although it might easily fly away. This is an old experiment which was studied by the celebrated Jesuit Athanasius Kirchner, professor in the Roman College, who published a book in 1646 with the strange title of '*Ars magna lucis et umbræ.*' In the chapter '*De imaginatione gallinæ,*' he describes the following experiment: If the feet of a hen are tied together, and she is then laid upon the floor, she will at first try to free herself by moving her body and flapping her wings, but when she perceives that all attempts are vain, she remains quiet. If, as soon as she is motionless, a line is drawn on the floor with a piece of chalk, beginning near her eye, the bird will not try to escape even after the feet are loosed, nor even when she is coaxed to move.

Many of us, when boys, have captured a hen, screamed into her ear, and then, having put her head under her wing, have laid her breast upwards on the table, saying that she was asleep.

This trick, known I believe in many countries, may be considered as another form of the *experimentum mirabile* of Kirchner. No physiologist had occupied himself with this phenomenon until Czermak, in a treatise presented to the Academy of Sciences of Vienna in 1872, maintained that it arose from an hypnotic state, or momentary somnolence. But this hypothesis does not explain why the breathing is laboured, the eyes staring, why the animals are unable to move even when touched, nor why their comb and wittles are so pale, which is not the case in sleep.

Preyer was the first to declare that these effects are due to fright, and as there was no word in the German language expressing the condition of a man overcome with fright, who is incapable of speaking, moving, or thinking, he called it *cataplexy.*[30] From his work bearing this title I extract a few observations.

Of all mammals guinea-pigs are most susceptible to fright. Simply taking hold of them, and keeping them a moment in the hand without any pressure, is often sufficient to paralyse them with fear. Guinea-pigs may remain half an hour in this state, rabbits not more than ten minutes, while frogs will remain for hours without moving. It is impossible that this interval be spent in sleep, for the animals expel fæces and urine. Kirchner maintained the necessity of drawing a white line from the beak of

---

[29] Brehm: *Thierleben*, vol. iii. 1883, p. 601.

[30] From [Greek: kataplêx], [Greek: êgos], frightened.

the animal, so that it should imagine itself bound by this mark; but this is not true, as they remain just as motionless without the line, and cataplexy is even more easily produced when the animal sees nothing. Crabs taken out of the water allow themselves to be put into the strangest positions, and remain for a long time motionless. Preyer made similar experiments on frogs and mice.[31] Some serpents remain rigid when their head is slightly pressed, as Moses is said to have done before Pharaoh.

To produce this state a sudden, unexpected agitation is necessary; it is a matter of indifference in what way the animal is treated, as all depends on the violent fright caused. A similar condition has been observed in men struck by lightning and in animals after electrical discharges from a powerful machine. Many birds, though scarcely wounded by small shot, fall to the ground as though struck by lightning, panting, with wide-open eyes, and remaining motionless when placed on their back. This also is an instance of the cataplectic condition, for, as their wound is not mortal, nor even serious, they recover soon afterwards.

Some animals and many insects remain for a long time motionless when danger threatens. To one of these zoologists have given the name of *anobium*, as though it feigned death when touched. Many other coleoptera act in the same way, not even moving when they are caught, transfixed with a pin, and roasted over a flame. Preyer justly remarks that this cannot be a feint, nor an instinct which tells them to preserve the appearance of death as a means of saving their life; for it would then be incomprehensible that they should let themselves be burnt alive rather than abandon the deception.

Certainly an animal that does not move can more easily escape from an enemy. Darwin remarks that when an animal is alarmed, it stops an instant to collect its senses and discover the source of the danger, and decide whether it should escape or defend itself; but this is certainly not the origin and reason of the phenomena of cataplexy and fear, which we must consider as a serious imperfection in the animal organism.

The phenomena which we are at present investigating find a counterpart in the story of the Medusa petrifying those who looked upon her, in the legend of the basilisk that could kill with a look, and of the serpent that caused death to mortals by hissing. One of these legends holds its ground to the present day, namely, that the breath of serpents is poisonous, and that they have a magic power in their look which attracts and fascinates their prey. But this is not correct, these also are cataplectic phenomena. When defenceless birds see a serpent approach their nest, they begin to scream and flap their wings, as though trying to draw its attention upon themselves, and so to save their young. Blinded by love and emotion they rush upon the enemy

---

[31] W. Preyer: *Die Kataplexie.* Jena, 1878.

and then remain as though paralysed, scarcely moving wings or claws, or else they let themselves fall into the jaws of the serpent and are devoured.

IV

It is well-known that fear may result in sudden death. Bichat maintained that it was essentially paralysis of the heart which causes death in strong emotions. 'The forces of the circulatory system,' he says, 'are worked up to such a pitch that they cannot recover from the sudden exhaustion, and death ensues.'

Old people in particular are liable to succumb to strong mental emotions. This fact stands in apparent contradiction to that of their sensibility, which is generally much less acute than in youth, but it is the weakness of their nervous system which destroys the balance. Often after great catastrophes parents succumb in consequence of the death of their children, while the brothers and sisters offer more resistance to grief.

Marcello Donato and Paolo Giovio relate that at the siege of Buda, in the war against the Turks, there was a youth whose valour excited the admiration of all. Unhappily he fell a victim to the repeated attacks of the besiegers. When the battle was over, the leaders hastened to learn who the hero was. Scarcely had the visor been taken from his face than Raischach of Swabia recognised his son. He stood motionless, his eyes fixed upon his son, then fell dead to the ground without uttering a word.

As a proof that weakness more easily causes death in emotion, I here mention an experiment of Johannes Müller. He destroyed the liver of some frogs, thus rendering them very weak and excitable. The slightest stimuli produced contractions in them, but they did not move if left in peace, and even lived for a long time. Those he took into his hand were immediately attacked by tetanus and died in a few seconds.

Haller tells of a man who, in stepping over a grave, imagined himself seized by the foot, and died the same day; others have died from fear on the day predicted as the day of their death, and some have fallen down dead at the moment they were condemned to death. Haller had already noticed that fear could arrest the action of the heart and profoundly modify the circulation of the blood: *hæmorrhagias supprimit, et menses, et lac, viresque ad venerem necessarias frangit.*

Surgeons well know how fatal a violent shock to the nervous system from traumatic or moral causes may prove to their patients. In such cases the medulla oblongata is so depressed in its activity that chloroformisation is sufficient to arrest the action of the heart and respiration. Porta, the great surgeon of the University of Pavia, when his patients died under an operation, used to throw his knife and instruments contemptuously to the ground, and shout in a tone of reproach to the corpse: *'Cowards die from fear.'*

My friend Lauder Brunton, professor of medicine at the hospital of Saint Bartholomew, in London, published the following fact a few years ago.[32] An assistant had made himself odious to the students of a certain college; a body of them, therefore, resolved to give him a fright. They put ready a block and an axe in a dark room, then seized the man and led him before a few students dressed in black, who officiated as judges. When he saw these preparations he took it for a joke, but the students assured him that all was meant in earnest, and that he must prepare for death, for he should presently be beheaded. They bound his eyes, forced him to his knees, and bent his head on the block. While one of them made a noise by brandishing the axe, as though to strike the fatal blow, another struck his neck with a wet towel.

When they took the bandage from his eyes he was dead!

V

One of the greatest physiologists of fear was Edgar Allan Poe, the unhappy poet who lived in morbid hallucinations, and died at the age of thirty-seven in a hospital, a victim to intemperance, amidst the horrors and convulsions of *delirium tremens*.

No one has ever described fear more minutely, none have so ruthlessly analysed, or made us feel with more intensity, the pain of overwhelming emotions—the throbbing which seems to burst the heart and crush the soul, the suffocating oppression, the awful agony of him who awaits death. No one ever plunged the mind of man into more horrible abysses, or led it into darker, gloomier wildernesses. None have ever inspired such horror with storm, tempest, the phosphorescence of decay, the lightning-flashes in the dead of night, the sighs and moans losing themselves in the darkness, the grip of fleshless hands amid the mystery of graves and ruins.

Who can forget those midnight terrors, those streaks of lurid light, those faint footfalls in the dark which make us shudder, those murders which paralyse the limbs, the groans, the strangled cries from the depths of a soul in agony? And those pulsations of the heart, deep, rapid, restrained, sending forth, like a muffled bell, a dull sound which spreads in the silence of the night, beating, throbbing even after death? How useless becomes even the courage of despair before these motionless spectres which fill us with terror! And the tortures and horrors for which words fail us, which still the heart, close the staring eye and numb the trembling limbs, stretch us senseless on this rack of fright and kill us with agony!

---

[32] Lauder Brunton: *On the Pathology and Treatment of Shock and Syncope*, p. 8.

CHAPTER XV

MALADIES PRODUCED BY FEAR

I

Unhappy invalids who must seek shelter in the hospital, and drag themselves feebly through those long wards where quiet has reigned for centuries, only broken by the sobs and cries of those poor wretches who come to lie down within these walls, as in the common tomb of the homeless!

How depressed they are when they leave their family and note the sadness of the place, advance sighing towards an unfamiliar bed, while around them they see all the ills which misery begets, and breathe the oppressive air of that pity which has gathered them together!

The new-comers at once recognise those more dangerously ill, even though they are at some distance, because the physicians stay longer beside them, watching them, the assistants and nurses are occupied with them. Then the bell for the viaticum rings; all who are able rise to their feet; then the extreme unction—then the rattling in the throat in the death-agony. And when at last they see the curtains drawn around the bed, a low, trembling whisper passes the sad news from mouth to mouth, to the most remote corners of the ward, beyond the dim rays of the funeral torch shining in the night like the last flicker of life in a body waxing cold for ever.

In their morning round the physicians find that the serious cases have grown worse, while those who are better beg to be dismissed. But it is in the women's ward that similar sad circumstances cause the most alarming effects. The physician who has the night-watch must walk up and down the whole night, prescribing soothing draughts and cordials, without his presence or his words of comfort preventing convulsive attacks or fainting fits.

Many patients die in the hospitals from fear and depression who would probably have recovered had they been tended in their own homes.

We must hope that thrift may so increase that the poorest working-man may have a cleanly house in which he may be nursed by his family when he falls ill, and that public benevolence may erect modest houses for those unhappy ones in need of succour, where the patient may enjoy efficacious scientific aid, and those comforts which the advance of hygiene demands, and be spared the heart-rending sights and injurious effects of the old hospitals.

II

The young physician, just beginning to practise, is astonished at the remarkable things which his patients tell him with the utmost confidence and in all good faith.

Nearly all relate the story of their illness, beginning with that circumstance which, in their opinion, originated it. It is an innate tendency which spurs the human mind to find an explanation for everything; and the reason of phenomena, which is the foundation of science, is yet the cause of prejudices and the most abundant source of error. If I were to mention the names of all the maladies which are thought to be produced by fear, I should be obliged to copy nearly the whole index of a pathological text-book, and with small advantage to the reader, for the authors, after exhausting their scientific matter, state empirically everything their patients tell them, provided their affirmations bear an appearance of truth. I shall only mention facts beyond doubt, or those least controversial, supporting them by examples taken from the most reputed authors.

Chomel relates that a physician, after having performed the autopsy of a man who had died from hydrophobia, was so overcome by the fear of having infected himself, that he lost both appetite and sleep, felt a horror of all liquids and a choking sensation in the throat when he forced himself to drink. For three days he wandered through the streets like one desperate. His colleagues and friends, believing it to be the effect of imagination, made every effort to convince him of the fact, and by keeping him with them, they succeeded in ridding him of the ill-omened thought, and he recovered.

It is an incomprehensible phenomenon, but yet admitted by all medical writers, that fear may of itself give rise to phenomena exactly resembling those of hydrophobic infection. A celebrated physician, Bosquillon, believed that fear alone was the cause of hydrophobia and not the bite or the saliva of the dog.

Dubois tells of two brothers who were bitten by a mad dog. One had to leave at once for America, and thought no more about it. When he returned twenty years afterwards, he heard through some thoughtless person that his brother had died of hydrophobia, and was so agitated by the news that he fell ill and died, showing all the symptoms of rabies. Medical works are full of instances of persons bitten by dogs, who only developed hydrophobic symptoms after being incautiously told that the dog was mad. It is often impossible even for the physician to distinguish hypochondriac hydrophobia from true rabies; even the manner of death is no guide, for tetanic contractions of the respiratory organs appear also in hypochondriac hydrophobia.

The physician can often save these patients, if he knows how to exert authority and to make use of means to convince the sufferer that he has nothing to fear.

The story is told of a physician who was called to a female patient infected with actual rabies, after his colleagues had declared that she was incurable. He examined her attentively, then kissed her on the mouth to prove to her that she was not hydrophobic. The patient recovered.

More especially during epidemics does fear play havoc. From the most remote antiquity physicians have observed that the timid die more easily. Giorgio Baglivi, in his celebrated book 'Praxis Medica,[33] describing the effects of an earthquake which took place in Rome in 1703, says that although not a single person was killed, several died of fever through fear, many women miscarried, and all bedridden invalids grew worse. Larrey had already noticed that on the fields of battle and in the lazarets soldiers belonging to the conquered army succumbed more easily to their wounds, while the victors more speedily recovered. This was confirmed in the war of 1870.

Fear alone may develop all the symptoms of a pestilential malady, even when the epidemic causes are totally wanting. Just recently, in one of his works on hysteria and hypochondria, Jolly relates the case of a patient of his, a lady in Strasburg, who received the news of the death of a relative from cholera in a distant country. She was very much frightened, and imagined that she herself was attacked by it. She lost her appetite and suffered for eight days from violent attacks of diarrhœa, and only after convincing her that there was not a single case of cholera in Strasburg, and that she was a prey to her own imagination, was it possible to allay the serious intestinal disturbances produced by fear. As soon as a report of cholera spreads through a town, all hypochondriacs feel worse.

Physicians who have described the dreadful spectacle of the lazarets during epidemics, mention the great number who die victims to fear, in many of whom the symptoms of the plague had not even appeared. Some have died suddenly from the fear of being taken to the lazaret, others have committed suicide, as we are told the cowardly have been seen to do in battle, who, terrified at the sight of death, or weary of suffering, have placed their chin on the muzzle of their gun and blown out their brains.

What horror we should feel could we read year by year the story of those who have succumbed to nostalgia, grief, humiliation; in misery, winter-cold, or want of food! Of men who have died hopelessly in the snow or lost in the sands of the desert, of others who have been shipwrecked and thrown upon the rocks, and whom a little courage might have saved; of men who have languished in gloomy prisons, in lonely monasteries or in exile, and who have died rather of mental than of bodily suffering.

III

Maladies which have their origin in fear must be distinguished from those morbid conditions which are suddenly aggravated by the effect of a strong emotion.

There are many who, when they receive a fright, become for the first time aware of some infirmity, which then increases so rapidly as to endanger their life.

Lamarre tells the following fact.[34] A lady, seventy-five years of age, had suffered for about ten years from defective action of the valves of the heart without this disease

---

[33] Baglivi: *Praxis Medica*, liber. i, cap. xiv. s. 5.

[34] Ed. Lamarre: *Contribution à l'étude du rôle du système nerveux dans les affections du cœur.* Paris, 1882, p. 99.

134

having hindered her housewifely activity. Dr. Lamarre, who was her physician from 1865 to 1870, was called a few times to her. The hypertrophy of the heart sufficiently counterbalanced the defect of the valves, and the pulse was regular.

When the Franco-Prussian war broke out in 1870, her sons agreed to keep her in ignorance of it, lest she should be afraid, she having already witnessed the plundering of her father's house by the Prussians in 1815. They succeeded easily in keeping all news of national disasters from her, for they lived isolated in the country, and their mother read no newspapers.

On September 4, 1870, she suddenly heard of the defeats of the French, and of the march of the German army upon Paris. It was such a terrible shock to her that her face became livid, and she scarcely had the strength to cry, as she pressed her hand to her heart, 'I am suffocating—I am suffocating!' Three-quarters of an hour later she died in her sons' arms.

The movements which she made with hands and face till the last moment, and the great irregularity of the pulse, caused Dr. Lamarre to abandon the idea of apoplexy, and accept as the cause of decease a nervous perturbation of the heart brought on by violent mental agitation.

Pinel, one of the greatest celebrities in the domain of mental diseases, always began the examination of a patient by asking him whether he had not had some fright or some great vexation. In the study of every nervous malady great importance must always be attributed to the investigation of the moral causes. The vivid impression of a strong emotion may produce the same effects as a blow on the head or some physical shock. There are men who, through fear, have lost consciousness, sight, or speech; others, still more sensitive, have remained for a long time paralytic, unable to move legs or arms, and have lost all sensibility. Some remain for a long time sleepless, others fall into a sort of exaltation resembling the outbreak of mental disease, many lose their appetite, or are afflicted with articular diseases, and in some the nervous system suffers such a shock as to cause violent fever.

Dr. Kohts, in his account of the maladies caused by fright during the siege of Strasburg in 1870, gives a minute description of the cases of *paralysis agitans* and of convulsions which he observed. The tremor and singing in the ears arose suddenly, often lasting for months, and even for life in very nervous persons, as is also the case in catalepsy, paralysis, and aphasy.

Leyden considers fright as one cause of myelitis. Likewise, in sclerosis of the arteries, cardiac hypertrophy, fright may produce hemiplegy. Berger instances two cases of perfectly healthy persons who, immediately after a fright, were attacked by paraplegy, with accompanying insensibility, without any serious anatomical injury, for the phenomena rapidly disappeared.

It is often said, and with good reason, that children should not be allowed to witness an epileptic fit, for the fright and emotion which they suffer may prove dangerous, causing later a similar attack in themselves. However difficult it may be to comprehend such a thing, it is yet admitted by all. Quite recently Eulenburg and Berger saw two old men, the one seventy, the other sixty-five years of age, who had an epileptic fit immediately after such a fright, although they had never had one before, nor were they predisposed to it. Romberg gives an instance of a boy, ten years old, who was frightened in the morning by a dog, and in the evening had an attack of St. Vitus's dance.

One of the most moving instances I have read about the influence of fear on the organism is in the description of the voyage of a sailing ship, so storm-tossed that one wonders how it could withstand the hurricanes which burst upon it. When scurvy broke out on board, the doctor noticed that the disease increased whenever the fear gained ground that land might still be far off. In every fresh tempest several died, and others were seized with the malady; and when at length the captain died, in whom all had great faith, the number of patients became five times greater.

IV

The passions have been divided by physicians into the exciting and the depressing. This distinction cannot, I think, be maintained at the present day, for we need only think of the effects we see produced by fear to be convinced that this emotion, which may at first appear exciting, becomes instead depressing in its paroxysms. The same may be said of narcotics and depressive remedies, which, in small doses, excite, but in larger doses depress.

Some phenomena, such as the growing grey of the hair, the immediate transmission of a nervous malady from the mother to the fœtus under the influence of fright, the possible death of sucklings a few hours after the mother has suffered great fear, although the infant was not present—all these are incomprehensible phenomena which we only admit because trustworthy observers and physicians affirm that they have witnessed them.

Michea, a celebrated physician, one of the most profound in knowledge of mental diseases, used to write insulting anonymous letters to some of his patients in order to cure them, and, he assures, with good result in some hypochondriacal cases. The mind may be drawn off from a fixed idea by preoccupying it with some danger. Physicians have sometimes had recourse in hysterical cases to threats or a sudden fright to check dangerous symptoms when all other remedies have proved useless. Amann tells of an hysterical patient who suffered from tetanic convulsions and trances, and whose father treated her with blows and cured her.

It is a well-known fact that fear sobers the drunken and cures slight nervous affections, but nothing can encourage the physician to raise fear to the rank of a curative method, as it may be expected that in the greater number of cases nervous diseases would be aggravated by such treatment.

Less questionable is, perhaps, the efficacy of fear in subduing nervous maladies acquired by simple imitation; in this case it is probable that the greater ill, as the saying is, drives out the lesser. In old books of medicine stories are found of psychic maladies which, under the name of St. Vitus's dance, or tarantism, affected entire provinces with a morbid excitement. The first symptoms of this malady appeared in Aix-la-Chapelle, then it broke out in Cologne, afterwards in Metz, whence it spread along the Rhine. Artisans, peasants, rich and poor, in hundreds left their families, dominated by an irresistible desire to dance. Intoxicated with excitement, they performed frenzied contortions as though possessed, until at last they sank exhausted to the ground or became incurably insane.

In suchlike cases Boerhave had recourse without hesitation to fright and violent emotion to prevent the patients giving way to their inclination. The story is told that while he was physician of the orphan asylum in Haarlem, he suppressed an epileptic epidemic by means of fright. Seeing that epileptic fits were daily increasing among his patients, he ordered a large brasier full of coals to be lighted in the room, heated a number of pincers and tweezers red-hot, and then told his little patients he had given orders that all those who had fits should be burnt.

This inhuman method gave rise to repulsive applications in the treatment of epilepsy, but cases of cure resulting are so exceptional that they certainly do not counterbalance the aggravated sufferings of those uselessly subjected to a cruel emotion. This notion, that maladies produced by strong emotions may be cured by others equally strong, is found in the oldest books on medicine. Pliny relates that the blood of the gladiators used to be drunk as a cure for the falling-sickness.[35]

We read miraculous stories of persons who suddenly became dumb, and of others who have regained their speech; and, indeed, such occurrences take place still, although they lose the dignity of the miraculous as soon as they are studied in the infirmaries.

The following is a case recently described by Dr. Werner.[36] A girl, thirteen years old, suffered a great fright by falling under a carriage. She escaped with a slight scratch, but suddenly lost her speech. Dr. Werner tried to cure her by various methods during thirteen months, without any result. At last he had prescribed bromide of potassium, when one day the girl threw herself into her mother's arms and said, in a laboured voice, 'Mamma, I shall speak again.' After one week she spoke as before.

Wiedemeister tells a story of a bride who, as she was taking leave after the wedding breakfast, suddenly lost her speech and remained dumb for several years, until, overcome with fear at the sight of a fire, she cried out 'Fire! Fire!' and from that time continued to speak.

Pausanias, too, relates that a youth recovered his speech in the fright caused by the sight of a lion, and Herodotus, in his history, narrates that the son of Crœsus was

---

[35] Plinii *Historia Naturalis.* 'Sanguinem quoque gladiatorum bibunt, ut viventibus poculis, comitiales morbi; quod spectare facientes in eadem arena feras quoque horror est.' Lib. xxvii. p. 9, vol. viii.

[36] Kussmaul: *Die Störungen der Sprache*, p. 200.

dumb, and that, at the taking of Sardes, seeing a Persian with drawn sword about to kill his father, he cried out, overcome with fright, 'Kill not Crœsus!' and from that moment he was able to speak.

CHAPTER XVI

HEREDITARY TRANSMISSION. EDUCATION

I

The most difficult thing in the study of man is to surprise him on the threshold of life, to meet him as he detaches himself from the tissues of the mother, in the guise of a cell seeking the mysterious contact of the fertilising element; to seize the moment in which that wondrous force containing potentially the whole story of an existence penetrates the chemical elements of the germ; to learn how, in the protoplasm of the first imperceptible nucleus, that marvellous activity awakes which only death will end.

There is a comparatively long period at the very beginning of our existence in which the nature and differential properties of the tissues lie, so to speak, dormant in a crumb of protoplasm. Microscopists discover no difference between the cells of that primary tissue. The turbidness appearing on the whitish leaflet of the germ seems regulated from the beginning of the division of labour; at a few points the materials accumulate which are requisite for the transformation of the cells, as though these last, too much occupied in their prodigious activity of separating and multiplying, must find close at hand the materials which they need to make a man, without the delay of elaborating and preparing them before they introduce them into their body. Thus it has been found, that from the beginning sugar or glycogen, one of the most important substances in the composition of the muscles, is present in abundance.

But up to this point, and even for many days afterwards, there is no indication, no possible recognition, even of a rough outline of a human form. And yet in this confusion of atoms we exist. Here our passions lie sleeping; on this whitish leaflet are written in undecipherable characters those links of heredity which connect us with our family and with past generations. As from the scarcely visible germ in the heart of the acorn the majestic oak will spring to reign over the forest, so from this indistinct cellular mass a being will be formed to represent in his microcosm the whole history of the human race, with its fears, diseases, instincts, passions, its hate, vileness, and grandeur.

The terrible legend of curses blasting the innocence of unborn babes, the blessings cast forth into the future for the enjoyment of generations yet to come, are not wholly a foolish fable. Destiny loads each one of us with a fatal inheritance. Though we were abandoned in the forest, imprisoned in the dungeon of a tower, without a guide, without example, without light, there yet would awake in us, like a mysterious dream, the experience of our parents and our earliest ancestors.

What we call instinct is the voice of past generations reverberating like a distant echo in the cells of the nervous system. We feel the breath, the advice, the experience

139

of all men, from those who lived on acorns and struggled with the wild beasts, dying naked in the forests, down to the virtue and toil of our father, to the fear and love of our mother.

II

Methods of education are essentially two in number, severity and indulgence. Which is better? It is impossible to give a categorical answer, for we are not concerned with the education of a brain or a man in general, but of the brain and man of a special case.

Some say that until the child has become a rational being it must be considered and treated as a little animal, because it has no sense of shame, nor of the rights of property, nor of social duty; that the didactic methods which it most fears must be adopted, that is to say, those only which serve to tame and domesticate animals— punishments, the whip, blows.

Happily, in the midst of the animal instincts a light is soon diffused in the child's brain which will place him above all the animals of the earth, and none can say with certainty when these first flashes of reason appear.

The pain of a blow must always appear to him so out of proportion to all his instinctive, involuntary movements, that instead of softening him it will rouse profound resentment in him, and impress him with the distressing idea of permanently threatening dangers and of the strangeness of his surroundings, in which, without any plausible reason, caresses alternate with blows.

The same methods should be followed in education as in the teaching of science, which are those giving to man the firmest and most lasting convictions. Whatever may be the force of authority, it can never be compared in efficacy to that of conviction; we should never issue any command without showing the reasons why it should be done in this way rather than in another.

Children should be brought up as though they were rational, because the animal in them disappears, the man remains. Recourse should be had to the most intelligible and convincing means; if it is seen that they have acquired bad habits, the opportunities for ill-doing should be removed and the effort made, by offering them other attractions, to preserve them from the temptation of those acts or those things which they are to avoid.

One may be more indulgent with good, docile children. Those who cry easily, who blush and scream, give less trouble than those who grow pale and tremble, who do not manifest their resentment by an immediate outburst, as though they were brooding hatred in a corner of their hearts.

A peasant-woman, in speaking of someone, once said to me: 'I have seen him gnash his teeth when a boy for a mere nothing, and so I would not marry him, and I was quite right.' In mental sufferings, when the tension of the nervous system cannot find a vent in immediate emotion, it accumulates and becomes more incontrollable in long-suppressed outbursts; the rage which we thought subdued continues to torture us and gnaw our vitals.

Indulgence should be shown to nervous children who suffer from convulsions, or are predisposed to such. One must be kind to them and not oppose their caprices with too much severity, unless they are actually insensate. Even loving punishment provokes an explosion of grief and nervous agitation in these unhappy children; every violent emotion leaves an imperceptible, morbid, accumulative tendency behind. In opposing them one falls 'out of the frying-pan into the fire.'

It is better to preserve their lives and postpone stricter education till they become less sensitive; in the meantime they must not be fatigued with study, but strengthened like a plant which one places in the sun and open air, and from which one prunes the injurious shoots at a later time. This is often successful, and then they may be ranked again with healthy children. Even for the latter, premature education is a very grievous error. Parents who make their children learn too many things, sacrifice their future to gratify their own ambition. Nature must not be forced, nor the activity of the nervous system exhausted before the body has grown strong.

Parents who have already some weak spot—a little fault in the character, a slight blemish in the organism—should redouble their care in order to cure their children from their own defects. Just as a scirrhus, cancer, consumption, neurosis, are transmitted from one generation to another, just as the large mouth, the long nose, the eyes and hair of this or that colour, are inherited, so vices, virtues, and moral dispositions are handed down from family to family. In little villages especially, in which one may best trace the customs of an ancestor in the whole of his descendants, one often hears such sayings as 'His father was just the same; his grandfather was a great good-for-nothing, too.' 'Generosity is hereditary in that house.' Thus were cynicism and cruelty transmitted from one to another in the family of the Claudii.

The root of a family tree may be compared to one of those Chinese boxes full of other boxes gradually decreasing in size, the unending succession of which strikes us with wonder. Marriage and intermarriage with other families mix and mingle these boxes in such a way that an inextricable confusion arises; but if from some height we could watch the long line of generations, we should see that they continue slowly to disclose themselves. Some children resemble the grandfather, the great-grandfather, or the great-great-grandfather, as though a seed had passed through several generations without unclosing, and then had suddenly sprung into life with such resemblance in features, manners, voice, eyes, character, that the old people recognise it and say, 'He is the very image of his grandfather.' Thus the forefathers are born and live again in future generations.

III

What a wonderful phenomenon is this power in man to reappear in future generations by means of heredity, to transmit his own nature to his descendants by transfusing it—working it into their organism! And no less wonderful is it to see how not only instincts but organs gradually disappear in the course of generations when they are not put into action. In insects, crustaceans, fish, amphibians which have migrated to caverns and have lived for many generations in the dark, the eyes are almost imperceptible, and this is certainly not the result of natural selection, for eyes are not injurious even to beings living in the dark, but solely because, with the cessation of the activity of an organ, it must of necessity retrograde.

Three or four generations are necessary before horses completely lose their wild instincts, so that some horse-breeders only choose those that have been already trained in the circus.

If one takes two hounds exactly alike (of the same mother and the same litter) and accustoms the one to the chase, the other to watch the house; if one then allows them to breed separately, so as to form two distinct families, one to start the game for man when hunting, the other to guard his house against strangers, we may be certain that after four or five generations their instincts will be profoundly modified. If after ten years one takes a litter from each of these families descended from a common ancestor, and rears them in the same room under the same conditions, far from every noise, and brings them when they are grown into a meadow, it will be seen that, at the report of a gun, the offspring of the dogs trained for the chase will look around as though trying to espy a bird, while the others run off terrified.

On the shores of certain almost desert islands birds are found which, like the *Phalaropus* of Iceland,[37] are very much afraid of man, while those living in the interior of the island are not at all timorous. If one reads Brehm's 'Animal Life,' one finds similar instances of fear transmitted from generation to generation, with marked differences in the same species according to the relations which the animals have with man. Although monkeys in general are very timid, and always flee at the sight of man, the *Semnopithecus entellus*, which the Indians worship and honour as a divinity, has become so bold that it enters the gardens, steals everything, plunders the houses, rummages in the trunks and cupboards of the Europeans, and snatches food from off the table or out of their hands. A missionary relates that he was once in a disagreeable predicament, because he had nothing to offer to these impudent monkeys, and that, if he had not defended himself in time with a stick, the animals would have whipped him.[38]

---

[37] Preyer: *Kataplexie*, p. 107. 1878.

[38] Brehm: *Säugethiere*. 1883. Vol. i. p. 105.

The mechanism by which these far-reaching changes in the instincts of animals are accomplished and transmitted by means of heredity to successive generations is one of the most obscure facts in medicine. The drunkard begets children predisposed to madness, just as the syphilitic transmit their curse to the innocent victims to whom they give life, but we know nothing of the manner of transmission; heredity of instinct remains inscrutable; the physiologist cannot yet confront such problems, so that he becomes a simple chronicler of the facts of which he does not know the laws, nor the intricate connecting threads.

Brown-Séquard tried to subject this problem to experimental study, and obtained results which surprised all physiologists. He observed that guinea-pigs in which he had severed the sciatic nerve produced epileptic offspring, and that the destruction in male or female of certain parts of the nerve-centres caused marked malformation in the ears and eyes of the progeny.

Pasteur found that the lambs of ewes that had been protected from a contagious malady called anthrax by inoculation with a diluted virus, were not attacked by this disease, and that even when inoculated with the active virus which would cause the death of other animals, they resisted it and did not succumb. This fact was confirmed by Toussaint and others.

There were, indeed, many indications in science which led to the idea of protecting from diseases by means of heredity. If small-pox does not rage as formerly, if the victims are no longer so numerous, and if even the unvaccinated recover more easily, it is because a modification of our organism has been brought about through heredity and inoculation. Whenever this disease appears in a district which was never before infected, it rages as violently as formerly. The same thing takes place when the inhabitants of a country where this disease is unknown come to a town in the air of which the germs are present in abundance. The eight Eskimos who were brought a short time ago to the Jardin d'Acclimatation in Paris all died of the small-pox.

It is a well-known fact that children of the same stock do not all resemble each other like stereotyped editions. Very often brothers and sisters, although they may have a striking physical resemblance to each other, show great difference of character; and what is of more importance to our study, these variations occur even though all the members of a family have been brought up in the same way.

It is with heredity as with certain chemical combinations arranged in kindred categories because of similarity of structure and composition, although one is noxious, the other beneficial, one poisonous, the other neutral. Even in twins joined together— there are several cases in the annals of medicine—in those also which I studied together with Professor Fubini, who are connected at the lower part of the trunk and have only two legs together, and who must certainly have always lived under the same conditions, there are yet profound differences of character.

We must therefore distinguish between the hereditary and the personal character, the characteristics of the family and those of the individual.

IV

The greater the advance of science, the greater should be the authority of the physician in education. All pedagogic systems deviating from natural means lead us into error and into morbid conditions of mind and body. Education should be conducted according to the laws of life, the needs of the organism, and the material interests of society.

The study of all that relates to the development of the intellectual faculties, the cure of aberrations of instinct and moral defects caused by the turbulence of the passions are problems so closely connected with phenomena of the physical order, that the physiologist and the physician should devote their attention to them as to a biological fact, as to the cure of a disease.

Unhappily, even considered from this point, the problem of education presents most serious difficulties. Some passions are incurable; others the body cannot resist, but wastes rapidly away under them, as under the fatal sway of a galloping consumption. The will does not suffice, for itself is only the result of the vitality of the organism, and of the greater or lesser resistance of which the nervous system feels itself capable.

The succession of causes and effects often forms an indissoluble circle which man cannot break with the simple force of his will. *Weakness produces fear, and fear produces weakness.* Here is a fatal revolution in the functions of the organism. Of what use are the arbitrary and imaginary distinctions philosophers have made in the functions of the mind, when they cannot be separated from those of the body? There are in life fatal cliffs, currents which we cannot stem, and which carry us to inevitable destruction.

Weakness increases excitability, excitability foments lasciviousness, and lasciviousness in its turn begets weakness. Here the functions of the organism are like a gaping whirlpool, like an avalanche moving onwards and dragging us to the fatal precipice, does a foot but slip on the path of life.

We now see that in our body some mechanism is lacking which would act as a curb to save us when we fall. It is one of the greatest imperfections of our nature that at every false step we may be thrown down and crushed, as though in the wheels of a machine. We may compare ourselves to those poor wretches who intoxicate themselves with opium or alcohol, and who, at last, cannot stop themselves on their downward path of intemperance, because if they cease drinking, opium-smoking, or opium-eating, there is an immediate aggravation of the morbid phenomena and tremor with which they are afflicted.

The primary cause of their disease now assuages the disease itself; it is a remedy which soothes them and slowly kills them.

Physiology is still too imperfect to make intelligible to us the intricate network of causes which impel man to act in one way rather than in another. Our eye cannot discern many important factors in human actions which, perhaps, will become evident to future generations. Chronicles, annals, biographies offer insufficient data and details too imperfectly known. I do not know when it will be possible to others to penetrate, as Taine did, far into the history of nations, to discover the biological laws governing the rise and fall of the greatness of a people. I only know that I am saddened and perplexed at the unhappy thought that, as the brain of the human race grows more perfect, the more sensitive and excitable will it become, the more will emotional desires wax within it.

V

Courage springs from three sources: nature, education, and conviction. Each of these may so preponderate as to compensate for the deficiency of the others. It is useless to say to a man, 'You must be courageous,' in order to make him so. Every day we see that the example of parents, education, admonitions, do not suffice to implant virtue in the children. There is a vital element in education which must be prepared long before, like the soil and the seed before the harvest; parents must bequeath to their children the inheritance of a constitution, robust and full of courage.

Fear attacks and nullifies every effort of the will in such a manner that it has always been esteemed a deed of heroism to combat and subdue it utterly. Alexander of Macedonia offered up sacrifices to Fear before he went to battle, and Tullus Hostilius erected temples and consecrated priests to it. In the museum of Turin there are two Roman medals, one of which bears the impression of a terrified woman, the other the head of a man with hair on end and frightened, staring eyes. They were struck by the consuls of the family of the Hostilii in remembrance of the vows made to propitiate Fear, which threatened to invade the ranks of the soldiers, who thereupon were led to victory.

The consciousness of strength makes us stronger. The history of medicine is full of the marvellous effects of confidence. If we were to cite all the examples of hysterical women, nervous, melancholy, paralytic men who, on the simple word of a physician, through faith in the efficacy of some remedy, have taken courage and recovered, we should see that every day wonders and miracles worthy of the saints are performed.

Neither may we say that it is all the effect of imagination, of fancy, because the modification of the circulation in the brain of one who resolutely determines to overcome a difficulty produces such an increase of energy in the nerve-centres and in the tension of the muscles that we sometimes see deeds performed by the pusillanimous such as were never expected of them, however strong and robust they may be physically.

We have seen that of itself the brain can originate nothing; at the most it seems to us free to choose amongst the various things presented to it. But, however heavily liberty may be fettered, it is yet beyond doubt that we may give a certain direction to our mind, and the aim of education must be to keep the attention continually fixed on those things which can strengthen the character.

In his celebrated book on the 'Passions of the Soul,' Descartes says,[39] '*Pour exerciter en soi la hardiesse, et ôter la peur, il ne suffit pas d'en avoir la volonté, mais il faut s'appliquer à considérer les raisons, les objets ou les exemples qui persuadent que le péril n'est pas grand; qu'il y a toujours plus de sûreté en la défense qu'en la fuite; qu'on aura de la gloire et de la joie d'avoir vaincu, au lieu qu'on ne peut attendre que du regret et de la honte d'avoir fui, et choses semblables.*'

VI.

What is most difficult in education is persistence; what is most efficacious is example. Severity is useless, perseverance it is which wins the day; there is nothing more harmful and fatal than inconstancy of purpose.

The paramount object of education should be to increase the strength of man, and to foster in him everything which conduces to life. Children whom parents teach to attribute too much importance to every little pain are thus predisposed to hypochondria. Sadness is a languor of the body, and we know by long experience that the melancholy and the timid oppose less resistance to diseases than others.[40]

In women one minute of intense fear produces far more frightful effects, and inflicts far more serious injuries, than in men, but the fault is ours, who have always considered the weakness of women a charm and an attraction; it is the fault of our erroneous system of education, which only seeks to develop the affections of the woman, neglecting what would be more efficacious—the creation of a strong character. We sometimes imagine that the most important branch of culture is that which we attain through education and study, that the progress of humanity is wholly represented by science, literature, works of art which are handed down from one generation to another; but in ourselves, our blood, there is a no less important factor. Civilisation has remoulded our nerve-centres; there is a culture which heredity transmits to the brain of our children; the supremacy of present generations depends upon the greater power in thinking, the greater skill in acting. The future and the power of a nation do not lie solely in its commerce, its science, or its army, but in the hearts of its citizens, the wombs of its mothers, the courage or cowardice of its sons.

---

[39] Descartes: *Les passions de l'âme.* Article xlv, Première partie.

[40] *Melancholici, qui natura sunt timidi et inconstantes, frequentius reliquos in morbos incidunt.* An old adage found in the most ancient books of medicine.

Let us remember that fear is a disease to be cured; the brave man may fail sometimes, but the coward fails always.

CPSIA information can be obtained
at www.ICGtesting.com
Printed in the USA
BVHW071155120919
558269BV00001B/191/P